the new rules of wellness

Transformational Stories from Health
Experts Who Lead from the Heart

House of Wellness Publishing

HOUSE OF WELLNESS
PUBLISHING

Disclaimer

All the information, techniques, skills, and concepts contained within this publication are of the nature of general comment only and are not in any way recommended as individual advice. The intent is to offer a variety of information to provide a wider range of choices now and in the future, recognising that we all have widely diverse circumstances and viewpoints. Should any reader choose to make use of the information contained herein, this is their decision and the author and publishers do not assume any responsibilities whatsoever under any condition or circumstances.

-⌇⌇⌇→

Foreword by Dr. Dee Hacking

Did you know butterflies can't see their own wings? Due to their field of vision and light spectrum abilities, they have completely different visual experiences than we do. They have many unique attributes, significantly with their spectral luminance sensitivities; they can see light as we can't, but there is a catch… they cannot see how magnificent and beautiful they are, but everyone else can.

Within Volume 2 of The New Rules of Wellness, you will meet 24 incredible authors who will take you on a journey into their self-illumination, where the common golden thread of connection is within the viewing. Noticing their wings, setbacks are organically unfolding as a comeback waiting to happen, where consistency is key, and enveloped in each tiny step is the energy that counts the most. Each softly spoken word to themselves accumulates more than many people may ever know—stepping into themselves and their energy and creating new rules for wellness. When they lost all of their excuses, they found results. It's immensely exciting to facilitate and catapult these inspirational individuals onto the global stage to share their genius zones, offering support and inspiration as an example to you and your authentic self– to embrace all YOU bring into this life.

An old friend recently gave me a box of KIND Affirmation cards. My close-knit circle of peeps all know I love my morning affirmations routine, and I have considered myself both a learned and grateful individual, and I find myself still getting surprised by what messages come my way.

'You have no cause for anything but gratitude and joy,' echoed the Buddhist teaching on the card. The card is correct; the energy behind *NO CAUSE FOR ANYTHING BUT* moved me. What a great prefix! I whispered to myself, 'No cause for anything but… MAGIC in my day-to-day, I made it so that day and continue to do so, adding a new suffix daily.

At times in our lives, even in our everyday schedule, are feelings of confusion, and overwhelm. Mental panic may quickly and unexpectedly rise to the surface, and we find ourselves looking for a way *out* of a situation (or the case of a reoccurring thought track) that occurs to each of us.

I asked Life, 'Why can you be so complicated? '

Life said, 'Because people do not appreciate easy streets, you must experience and perceive it. Feel it, Live it. Experience it.'

I replied, 'Then, how did I become such a sad trainwreck a times—I'm tired and stressed, and this is not where I want to be in life?"

Life said with gusto, 'You will always have problems and conflicts of different kinds in your life; you must learn to enjoy life while solving them and to see your beauty while doing so.'

I feel there is a better way to become unstoppable and how to leave your mark on the world: It's about dancing in the rain, admiring the storm, having a down day, resting calmly, wiggling your toes in the wet grass, and maturing to value yourself. There is beauty in all things around us. It is time to adjust your perception and evolve, creating new rules around your living, health, and journey and assisting others through their journeys.

Become the person who thrives through shocking moments and unsupportive thoughts, succeeds through diversity, and offers solace to others.

In The New Rules of Wellness Volume 2, you will find "I can and I will" people and "I'm finding my way" people. "I'm doing my best, one day at a time, one moment at a time, I won't give up" people doing fantastic work in their fields. Actions fueled by self-will and embracing what comes their way. Each Author has found a way to make the most of each day, not lamenting the past or worrying about the future but somehow managing to make the most of each day. I'm delighted to support my Authors in my previous Volume 1 to become International Bestselling Authors in 2023, to showcase their journeys and work, and to support them all in continuing to share their energy cemented in that volume. I am now proudly a four-time International Bestselling Author and an International best-selling boutique Publisher, business owner, Homoeopathic Physician, and Clinician. I'm excited to do the same for my Volume 2 authors and watch them fly into their sparkling futures.

It's via conscious and intentional living, exploring issues, having an opinion, sharing experiences, talking of their failures, celebrating successes, finding opportunities to contribute to society, yes–creating ripples and waves, creating awareness, experiencing happiness and sadness, embedded struggles and conflict—then evolving. Learning, finding self-education, creating profitable ventures, and even non-profitable ventures, failure ventures, offering community support, communication with others, problem-solving, looking for ideas, that we can then be balanced, happy, and the ones who are serving others, being inspired, and in turn inspiring others too.

Reach out to me if you, too, would like to be featured in The New Rules of Wellness book series or dream of becoming a published solo author to share your thoughts, ideas, and opinions, especially if you find yourself saying '*I want to be the author of my narrative.*'

Who are you, and how will you leave your mark? How will you amplify your voice? Create impact? How will you see yourself, *see* your own wings? To think, feel, imagine, create, evolve, become—some heavy stuff, right? You've got this- DO IT anyway, regardless of your circumstances! Watch your life change when your only task is to make peace with yourself.

Even the softest voice and the loudest unspoken opinions are valued even in the smallest forms, encouraging passions to create books as a legacy, cultivating courage, and pushing the boundaries to become unstoppable.

It's time to call energy back to yourself. Remove all the costumes you have worn, expand your gorgeous wings, and perceive life differently, with no cause for anything but MAGIC!

Dr. Nereda (Dee) Hacking. House of Wellness Publishing
Ph.D.BHMS.B.Sc.Adv, Dip.Hom.Adv.Dip.RT
houseofwellnesspublishing@gmail.com

'*Peace comes from within. Do not seek it without.*'
~ W. E. Channing.

Contents

-⌁⌁➔

Dr. Dee Hacking

'Some people want it to happen; some people wish it would, and others make it happen.' ~ Michael Jordan

You are doing better than you think you are. You were different only twelve months ago; twelve months from now, you will be different again. I feel it's a kind of rolling and dynamic twelve-month cycle, and I find it amazing we can adjust our filter on the action taken: wanting, wishing, or making certain things happen...or not. People over the years tell me I'm blessed or lucky, I chuckle inside– *lucky? No, it's hard work and self-realisation too!* I'm a 'the show must go on' and 'believe,' even a 'self-love gal'!

I love the line: The presence of love is the absence of judgement. Those two things cannot hold the same space; everything you need is within you, and more will follow where you place your focus and energy. I keep an old photo of myself on my phone, a photo of me wearing a gorgeous outfit and a bonnet my mother made me when I was about three years old. I'm standing under a loaded Lemon tree with a broad smile. I tell the photo,

"It's OK, you make it. We've got this. You are amazing, and I love you."

Powerful, try it! So, I ask you this question: what are you creating in life and within yourself?

"You aren't going to go crazy," I said firmly in the bathroom mirror. "You're stronger than you think."

I sighed, expressionless. I watched my chest rise and fall with deep breaths, and my long red hair flowed over my shoulders like a warm hug. Was I wanting and wishing? Was I looking into my reflection, asking for help, and willing things to happen as I did as a child? My belief was so untamable I could see my vision all unfolding in the mirror before me, like wings expanding. Wishing and wanting are amazing, but forging out the steps and *making it all happen* is the magic. Believe, Believe, Believe—play the game of brief. Summon the *belief*, Genie! Act as you believe it, think as you believe it, and exist as you have already achieved it, that is power—that is sheer power. More powerful than wanting, willing, and wishing for sure.

Yet, twelve months ago, I felt like I was in a holding pattern. The moment I decided not to *think* myself into a doomsday scenario and to make the most of each thought– find a miracle in each moment, to make the most of each day in the best possible way (not what others wanted from me came to a huge realization – instead, what *I COULD* manage, what I WANTED to manage), my life changed.

I was doing so much better than I thought– I was smashing goals and *killing it.*

Yet, in a quiet moment, I wasn't 'performing' as my mind visualised. I had a big mental list of all the things I hadn't accomplished in my day, a little splice of grief there, too, for not completing my self-imposed duties, and the list grew. AND YES, I had it all in life, and I was hungry for it, inspired for it, passionate for it, and others were relying on me for it; people looked up to me for it and needed guidance from me for it, too, yet I felt in my soul disappointed for it that I was *slowly* getting there. SLOWLY > I stop myself in time. These repeating patterns weren't serving me well. The words in my mind were 'drawn out, and, of the secret space of my mind, and not performing so well.' But to visualise and VOICE these *lazy-non-performing thoughts* sounded ridiculous, so a chant emerged from my lips ...."I'm doing better than I thought I was," and my results soon matched my anointed title– *Killing it* and *Smashing it.* I'm excited and inspired to imagine twelve months from now!

I repeatedly stand in front of the mirror. (You know I have many friends and patients who haven't looked at themselves in the mirror for years?) "Goodness, NO, I don't look in mirrors, I hate myself!". We were participating in a group Personal Development Activity at a weekend seminar a few years ago, and we were to look into the mirror each morning and repeat our daily affirmations to our reflection. I LOVE this exercise, so many in the group not only found it difficult but were truly traumatized to view themselves.

"You aren't going to go crazy," I said firmly in the bathroom mirror. "You're stronger than you think. You are guided throughout this day and take supportive actions. Divine intelligence guides you."

I sighed. I smiled at myself. I watched my chest rise and fall with deep breaths, and my long red hair flowed over my shoulders like a warm hug— again, but smiling and feeling whole.

I continued, "The next time you feel that way, find something to focus on to remind you of who you are, your beauty, strength, and uniqueness."

I looked at my reflection deeply for signs of inner life. I look deeper. I see my unique talents; I see *love* flowing through me, I see my *belief* expression. I see a Blue Butterfly.

"Ahhhh, YES, a big Blue Ulysses Butterfly!" I smiled in the mirror and visualized her beautiful wingspan, the iridescent electric blue, and the subtle black. Her shiny black antennae and jet-black prolonged lobes at the end of her wings. I see her coming to rest on the back of my hand, and I can feel her little legs tickling the back of my hand. She closes her wings tightly as she rests on my hand, then gently unfolds them, exposing the magnificent blue coloring, and flies away in a darting motion.

The images have relaxed and calmed me. *I'm doing better than I thought*, and I get to work in my Alpha Brainwave way, on point and ready to slay my duties at hand.

Following that inner voice that whispers to your spirit, not the one that continually yells at your ego, was golden for me to experience. Do what your future self needs you to do to brighten your way. This was the shift that changed my life twelve months ago. Looking past the human figure's reflection, what do you see in the mirror?

The absence of problems is a myth.

I love that both happiness in life and our health are not the absence of problems but the ability to deal with them—your thoughts and opinions on handling your situations and how you feel you're progressing. Being open to things being more effortless and more magical is a choice and a pathway. I wish I could inform my younger self of this point. Having my Electric

Blue Butterfly with me each time I need her, rather than anger, frustration, and illness arising from stress, is amazing. It's not the absence of the stress that has your pulse racing, pressure in your chest, and nausea; it's the ability to notice and keep triggers at bay. It would be amazing to send all your problems through a wormhole, wouldn't it? I have imagined that too. Going through hardships is a sign of change, growth, and learning to count on yourself. Seeking peace over pleasure, learning from your mistakes, and knowing everything will be okay, somehow. The lessons you struggle with will repeat themselves unless you learn from them.

The only competition is with the person who you were yesterday.

It is okay to be sad after making a decision; it does not mean you've made a bad decision, it just means you are feeling your emotions and now can decide to make it a happy one. If everything is made of energy, energy is neither created nor destroyed; it exists. All things already exist in an energetic and vibrational state. When you desire something, it already exists on an energetic plane. Recognizing this is the key. If you desire something, If you experience the energy of it, feel it, imagine experiencing it, you can feel the reality of what you want, then remain in that energy until you see it in your reality.

I found myself trying harder and counterintuitively experiencing a deeper kind of stress. I needed to be slower and just breathe, but I felt to slay the day, I had to perk up and be at a higher production level. Along my journey of growth, my one new rule of wellness is to prioritize self-care, good food, supportive food habits, physical activity, rest, and the 100-day commitment rule. I started to polish my commitment crystal ball (that would be amazing if one existed, wouldn't it?), and I love it when inspiration hit me: 100-day commitments. This got me out of my stress cycle.

After the first 100-day process and taking notes, consistencies arose: When I was tired, I previously tried to add stimulants to force myself to go on no matter what.? Yet, Rest and reboot was the only way. If you feel restless, go for a walk. If you feel like giving up, remember when you succeeded and re-celebrate that win. If you're overwhelmed, write it all down. If you are lost and alone, call a friend. If you feel anxious, make some fun plans for the future—plan them out, and then focus on the present moment. If you need to be 'more— list your achievements. If you feel so lethargic, you could just sleep all day or watch movies, exercise—stretch, walk, wall pilates, anything–just move!

These are the cheat codes, WOW moments.

If someone insults you, don't react, reply to them with a concerned and empathetic expression— Are you ok? Only a person suffering inside will insult others. (become immune to those insults). Good posture increases confidence. Be cautious of insults disguised as jokes. Our happiness and well-being are what matters. Wake up and look at everything fresh.

Being the best version of yourself, your integrity and character will shine through. You cannot control how others talk about you, their opinion of you, or how others see you. Let our actions speak for themselves. People aren't against you- they're for themselves. The most significant limitation is not doing what you want. Stay away from playing games with yourself. Remember that you can do the little things and don't settle for less. You may need to understand why certain things happen. However, there is a higher energy to the events in your life; the turmoil can be a blessing to be revealed. You spend a lot of time with yourself, why not make yourself interesting?

During a clinical appointment, a dear patient, Rebekah, stated, " No, I'm so boring I even hate myself for it, so why would anyone else love me and want to be with me?". While we were dealing with her back and knee problems and discussing treatment for her Gall and Liver, we chatted about her life a little deeper and what she does for fun and self-care. "I do nothing I want to do! I would love to get back to swimming and Yoga classes, learn cheesemaking, and do an online course".

"So what's keeping you from doing any of that?"

"Well, I don't get around to thinking about it too much, life is busy, work is hectic, and I'm always tried, and I don't believe I can do it, to be truthful."

Belief. There it is.

I held Rebekah accountable to message the Yoga teacher, find out the class schedule —*action*- and locate a pool she could visit once a week. Who provides the online course, and how much it costs—-some research.

"OH MY GOSH DEE," she called me the next morning. " You won't believe this—Yoga classes are held down my road at the community center twice a week at 7 pm, there is a heated pool also down the road behind the Post office complex, and my course is free currently due to a government funding scheme, now to set cheesemaking next month. TICK!"

One month later, in her follow-up appointment with me on ZOOM, She loves the changes of replacing potato chips with popcorn, physically shaping up and ordering new swimmers, has lots of newfound energy, and made some friends at the pool to go to coffee with at the cafe next door.

"People like me, Dr. Dee, I'm starting even to like myself!!" She winked and whispered. She has someone special in her life now and was away on a cheeky weekend. Hence, the virtual TeheHealth call today—*inspiration, belief, and action!* What makes you feel most alive? Time to give THAT a massage and nurture it, self-care the hell out of it! Herd in the bits and pieces that have you ALIVE!

I've made up a Good Life balance sheet and am now blasting it with sunshine. I have balance sheets for my business, why wouldn't I have one for my successes? I have a column for Family, Friends, and Fitness. I divide 24 hrs into 8 + 8 + 8; sleep, work, and 'life'. You can't start a new chapter if you keep reading the old ones—the column for Health, Hygiene, and my passion project. (Which currently is a book of my short stories, 'The Invisible Pyramid'—look out for that one in 2024!). The next column is Spirituality, Smile, Service; start running the Smile marathon. Service and giving back is vitally important to me. I've supported The Royal Flying Doctor service for over 30 years.

Life is complicated. As a Clinician, Publisher, Author, and problem solver, people ask me to find answers to their issues—asking and searching for answers is exhausting and unfulfilling as life then changes all the questions. There is a better way— to set intentions: you need a life filled with great times, happiness, and contentment and to feel clear, whole, and centered. What do you need to release, overcome, or let go of?

We all have a list that we mostly avoid and continue to complain about. What do you want in your life right now, what do you need to strive for, and what are you divinely guided toward? What keeps you up at night? What could you address today that may springboard you into a future you long for? Get in touch with that innate inner wisdom and get some separation from your past, old patterns, old opinions, and old thinking, and align more with your new desires. One minor step executed consistently will have you at a desired result naturally, organically, and with little effort, an imminent magical arrival.

What do YOU, yes, *YOU* in the mirror, need right now?

Me? I need a collagen face mask and sleep!

Another gorgeous patient of mine said the loss and trauma of her late husband both haunts and pains her daily. The trauma involved in not knowing WHY he was so ill for so many years, then ultimately WHY he died (until an autopsy was performed - then the answers revealed as a genetic influence).

"Though you are apart physically, spiritually, and energetically, there needs no separation; you are always united."

My words were met with a frown, and I'm sure she thought I was on a gradient of insanity until I explained. She then met me with a broad smile after just one of my Mystic Alpha Brainwave Sessions and a reply of *'an utterly relaxed state. The grief had lifted in its entirety, and she felt whole again. Nothing is missing. I feel him beside me, talking to me. I feel whole.'*

For love transcends space and time; it's all energy, we are all energy, and the universe is all energy within specific and varied densities and frequencies. Why are we not utilizing this as a personal rule for wellness, I certainly do, and have done so since I was 16 years old.

"I am rather taken aback," she states one day before her session. "Sometimes when I'm in the Alpha Brainwave state, and I have my husband sitting next to me on a large rock in a magnificent rainforest, with butterflies flying around us, the smell of sweet Orchids in bloom and the trickling of the stream beneath cooling our feet, I feel like I am eavesdropping on many years of conversations we had not yet had."

"Beautiful", I reply. "Grief and trauma cannot exist in a space of Joy and Happiness."

"Thank You, You've changed my life!"

We sat in silence. Smiling. Allowing peace.

No one is like you; It's OK to be you– be yourself and know yourself.

The life before you is far more important than the life behind you. Reach out to me and see how I can assist you best. This can be the magic of your health and wellness journey via confident, consistent choices and small actions, empowering you to live the life you love, a life you don't need to remediate or escape from. Are you waiting to *feel better*, have more money, or have more time so you can create the life you desire? Until you can spread your wings and SEE those beautiful wings, you will fly into the next amazing phase of your life and live a great life anyway.

Sprinkle some belief magic on it, and do what your future self needs you to do!

Dr. Nereda (Dee) Hacking
Ph.D.BHMS.B.Sc.Adv, Dip.Hom.Adv.Dip.R

***

Inspiration Anyway ~ Mother Teresa

People are often unreasonable, illogical, and self-centered; forgive them anyway.

If you are kind, People may accuse you of selfish, ulterior motives; Be kind anyway.

If you are successful, you will win some false friends and some true enemies; Succeed anyway.

If you are honest and frank, people may cheat you; Be honest and frank anyway.

What you spend years building, someone could destroy overnight; Build anyway.

If you find serenity and happiness, there may be jealousy; Be happy anyway.

The good you do today, people will often forget tomorrow; Do good anyway.

Give the world the best you have, and it may never be enough; Give the world the best you've got anyway.

You see, in the final analysis, it is between you and God; It was never between you and them anyway.

About the Author

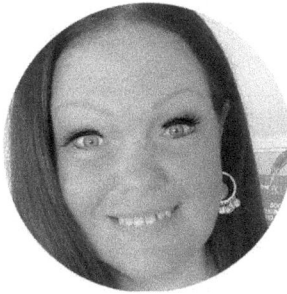

Dr. Dee Hacking is proudly the creator of The New Rules of Wellness book series, is an International bestselling boutique publisher, four times International Bestselling Author, Ghostwriter, and Homeopathic Physician obtaining her doctorate studies while running her busy clinic.

Dr. Dee hails from metropolitan Melbourne, Australia, and lives in tropical North Queensland, Australia, with her loving husband, John. Jointly, their three children, are spread across the globe living their best lives and when you don't find Dee in her favorite coffee shop, or swimming laps, or at the Warrior Gym, you will find her curled up in her reading- nook amongst her pile of books in her 'to be read next' pile. She wants you to know that breaks can be mended, pains can be healed, and no matter how dark it gets along the way, the Sun will rise again and again; 365 new chances for Joy.

Email: houseofwellnesspublishing@gmail.com
Facebook: www.facebook.com/nereda.hacking
LinkedIn: Dr. Dee-Middendorp-Hacking

-wwww→

Ricky Adams

My New Rule of Wellness is the same as the old one: **Laughter is the best medicine.**

I laugh a lot. (Some might say too much, but there's no fun in listening to them!) There's so much in the world to laugh about. Laughter spreads joy and creates endorphins, those feel-good hormones that human brains love. Laughter can raise mood, show appreciation, lessen stress, bring people together. And all that just from the irregular passage of air in and out of our lungs! What a fantastic, powerful, and dare I say it – funny – thing.

The concept of "wellness" is something that everyone aspires to, one way or another. It's the road to that wellness that can be a very individual journey. With such a variety of tools and methods available, no two people's wellness paths would necessarily be anything alike. Everyone needs to find their own protocol. Some protocols will evolve and require a lot of modification, some will require restarts, and many will mean very hard work (ultimately, it is hoped, very rewarding work too). But do you know what is great about laughter as a tool to wellness? It's universal, it's free, and best of all, it's so EASY. No matter the "main" protocol to wellness you're following, a little simple laughter can go a long way – in concert with other rules of wellness, or all on its own.

Very few people are completely devoid of a sense of humour, with the possible exception of the man who was three seconds too late to stop his toddler flushing his brand-new iPhone down the toilet. Finding a way to laugh should be the easiest thing in the world, even if everything else seems hard. Laughing is also a very natural human thing, and is the one contagious thing that is actually good for us. So, find or create your laughter. Explore it, cherish it, nurture it, enjoy it, spread it, and most importantly, benefit from it. There's essentially no downside to trying it out, because laughing oneself to death is so very rare that the Wikipedia article about it (search "death from laughter" in Wikipedia) lists the "victims" by name (plus it sounds like they all had a great time on the way out!). And if you would like some tips for your Quest for Laughter? Please read on…

You don't have to be happy to laugh.

No one can deny that life is serious business. There's stuff going on in the world, and in our own individual lives, that can be a lot to take. Non-wellness is all around. Physical illness and mental illness require serious treatment. Laughter is certainly not the magic solution to life's problems. But if laughing helps, even a little, even if only for a little while, then that's a Very Good Thing. I took a break from writing this story because I received some bad news and needed to process it. And then later I didn't really feel like writing about laughter, but I do try to practise what I preach (and I wanted to feel even a little less shitty), so I went online to the website of a comic artist I like. I found myself laughing at one of my favourite comics (that I've laughed at many times before), and then I did feel less shitty. And I took a deep breath. And laughed at some more comics. And then moved on to something else, and something else, and now I'm writing this story again. You don't have to be happy to laugh, but if you can find something to laugh about, you may also find a bit of happiness as a result. And a little bit of happiness might be just what you need.

Learn to laugh at yourself.

Most people are afraid of embarrassing themselves. Well, everyone is going to embarrass themselves at some point in their life – that's just being human. We also share this space with other humans and animals, so even if you could magically avoid embarrassing yourself, someone or something else is bound to be kind enough to embarrass you, whether it's a malicious online troll or that bird who just couldn't wait until he'd flown completely past you before deciding it was toilet-time.

Ultimately, though, what does it really matter? Even if the worst-case scenario is that you end up looking foolish in someone's TikTok prank video that goes viral and then unflattering memes are made of you for years thereafter, eventually the heat-death of the universe will mean that no one will be around to remember or care – problem solved. The more you accept that your own existence is inherently fraught with opportunities for funny stuff to happen *to* you as well as *around* you, the easier it will be to laugh at yourself. And when you can laugh at yourself, you can defeat the fear of embarrassment, project a positive attitude (which benefits both you and those around you) and as a bonus, even find a kind of "cheat-code" to those sweet endorphins.

Remember that humour is subjective.

This is a really big one. All the time, people say, "That's not funny." What they really mean is that something isn't funny *to them*. Don't police another person's sense of humour – if you don't agree, leave it be. Likewise, don't let other people tell you what you should be finding funny or not – they're not you. Comedian Ricky Gervais has millions of fans around the world and has won awards for his TV shows and stand-up comedy specials. But there are many people who don't find his style funny. That doesn't mean he *isn't* funny, because "funny" is purely in the eye and ear and sensibilities of the beholder. If you like his type and content of comedy and you go to his live stand-up shows, you'll have a fantastic time, laugh lots, and enjoy the camaraderie of being with like-humoured people. But if you *don't* like Ricky Gervais, it's so easy just to ignore him, and find something or someone you *do* like. That's the beauty of humour – there are so very many kinds that something will resonate with anyone and everyone. Appreciating highbrow intellectual humour is just as valid as loving fart jokes or thinking that naming a ship "Boaty McBoatface" is the epitome of wit, if it appeals to you and produces that oh-so-beautiful laughter (and let no one smother it!). A lot of the fun can even be in the journey of finding just what works for YOU. The important thing is to find your laughter, and use it well.

Find your laughter everywhere.

To find what works to make *your* laughter, look everywhere! There are SO MANY THINGS in the world to laugh about, whether they just exist that way, or have been specifically contrived to promote laughter. The world is, frankly, absurd. For example, take animals. The way they look (aardvarks, leafy sea dragons, proboscis monkeys, red-lipped batfish, babirusas, shoebill storks – Google "weird looking animals" and you'll find these and so many more) and the way they behave (watch any wildlife series by Sir David Attenborough and see just how FUNNY as well as fascinating the world's creatures are). Whatever belief you subscribe to as to how the world got its animals, there's no denying that Mother Nature or the god(s) or the simulation's chief programmer had one bizarre sense of humour (as have a lot of the scientists who actually name the animals – "sarcastic fringehead" for a little brown fish is possibly my favourite). My point is, it doesn't take much to find something to laugh about in the world, even before you go looking for things that have been designed to try to make someone, somewhere, laugh. Cavemen may well have found stuff to laugh about but there were probably only so many jokes they could make about mammoths. Luckily for modern humans, we have TV, and even better, the internet. The internet is much more than just cats stealthily preparing for world domination or people redefining the word "fact" on social media. The internet contains a lot that is inadvertently humorous (news reports on practically everything politicians say or do, for example – lots of people laugh at those, especially when the alternative is to cry), but also so much stuff that has been created for the express purpose of eliciting laughter. There will be something for everyone, and there are so many websites devoted specifically to humour that fortunately it can take only the very minimum of effort to find something that works for you.

Cultivate your laughter to support your wellness.

This one is really, *really* important – in the context of this story, and for the point of this book. If you are utilising laughter in your pursuit of wellness, be mindful that *not all laughter is created equal.* There is positive laughter and there is negative laughter, and wellness wants to pitch its tent firmly in the "positive laughter" camp. Many years ago I was at a supermarket, waiting in a checkout queue. The supermarket was crowded. Only two self-checkouts were working, and their queues were longer than the one I was in for one of the two cashiered checkouts that were open. I had seven items, and I was fifth in line at the 15-item limit express checkout, and the four people in front of me all easily had more than 25 items each. I had nowhere else in particular that I needed to be, but you bet I was still wanting to get there fast, and I was very annoyed to be stuck in this supermarket queue instead, for No Good Reason. I was extremely grumpy. And then the customer currently being served, juggling his too-many items, dropped a big tub of yoghurt on the floor. The tub burst and splattered its contents across the floor and the customer's shoes. And for a second as I stared, knowing that this would mean further delay while the staff cleaned up, I had an urge to laugh at the customer with a "Serves you right!" attitude. However, the absurdity of the situation suddenly struck me, and I found myself chuckling instead at the universe humbling us all via yoghurt. My amusement grew as I noticed that one patch of yoghurt was making quite a rude shape on the floor (hurry with the mop there, staff member – there are young children in the queue!). I did hide my laughter as best I could so that the customer wouldn't actually think I was laughing at him, while I considered that as much as there's no point in crying over spilt milk, it certainly felt good to laugh over dropped fermented milk! And the "feeling good" part is my point, because from feeling grumpy and negative, I was now feeling happy and positive. A little light laughter, a little *right kind* of laughter, did wonders for my attitude that day, and for the future. That day I let the woman who was behind me in the queue, who only had two items and appeared as grumpy as I had been, go ahead of me once the queue was moving again. I had laughed and I felt better; the woman thanked me for letting her go ahead of me and perhaps she felt better; Mr Whoops-There-Goes-My-Yoghurt didn't see me laughing at all (he couldn't have known I wasn't laughing at him, had he seen me, because I don't think the yoghurt spill-shape looked quite as rude from his angle) and while that may not have made things better for him, it certainly didn't make them *worse*, and sometimes that's extremely important too. The best thing about the whole business for me was that not only did I have a much better rest of my day after The Yoghurt Incident, but I can honestly say that I have never been annoyed about waiting in a queue since. Before that day, I couldn't have imagined that just finding some childish humour in a food spill, and letting myself express that positively, could make such a difference to my attitude then and my spirit in the future. It was a wonderful thing to discover! I acknowledge that it may not always be that easy, not for everyone, and not all the time, but it's worth at least *trying* to condition yourself always to positive laughter, rather than negative laughter, and especially if you are actively looking to use laughter as a tool on your wellness journey. Laughing negatively at someone's misfortune, for instance, may have the same physical benefit as laughing for joy, but mental and emotional well*ness* (as important as physical wellness, if not more so on an individual basis) is best served from the mental and emotional well*being* that comes from positive experience with and of other living beings and the world. I find nothing so positive as a good laugh from joy, or cuteness, or a well-told joke, or the weird antics of an animal, or the wildly uninhibited things small children say (there are so many examples of those online, too!). And I have found that the more I cultivate positive laughter, the better the feedback loop, the better the wellbeing, and the more powerful the tool is for promoting or restoring wellness. I can't help but want to share that discovery, and I hope that a little of the experience and advice here and in the other tips might help someone else too.

So there you have it. Whatever else your wellness journey entails, maybe see if there is some room for a little positive laughter on the side, like a well-seasoned sauce that really brings out the flavour of the main dish. (That is actually a more palatable simile than laughter being like medicine, even if I do think it probably is still the best kind. And I am not just musing along those lines because it's dinner time as I write this...) The road to wellness may be full of rules, old and new, something for everyone. The wonderful thing is that laughter, as a rule (of wellness or otherwise), is for anyone.

About the Author

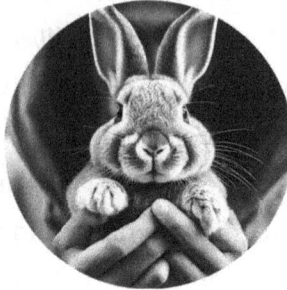

Ricky Adams is an Australian human who can laugh about just about anything. Including, but not limited to, being Australian. And a human.

Ricky has had many jobs and has travelled around many parts of the world. All of which only reinforces that there is something to laugh about everywhere, practically all the time.

Ricky loves stand-up comedy, especially that of Ricky Gervais (and not just for his name), Jim Jefferies, Sarah Millican, and Rita Rudner.

Ricky's absolute favourite animal is the rabbit, even though it really isn't as funny-looking as it could be.

Ricky lurks a lot on this subreddit

https://www.reddit.com/r/ContagiousLaughter/

-ᴡᴡᴡ→

Dr. Lorenzo Bianchi

Dolce far niente

My new rule of wellness: If you don't set some intentions for your wellness, no doubt you will be forced to take time out of your life for your illness.

The sweetness of doing nothing; Dolce far niente. Firstly, forgive me, English is my second language.

Dolce far niente; This is now me as I've retired and love sipping a light Prosecco in the Nepalese sunset, sometimes a Barolo if I feel like it. I have been an ALS all my life, a Physician who does Advanced Life Support with the Italian Paramedic's Emergency Services.

My wife and I have moved all over Italy in the past 30 years, we have also travelled worldwide on vacations and now decided to call Naples home. We have always loved the Southern Coast of

Italy—the contrast of old crumbling buildings, the food, the wine, and the amazing walking trails up Mount Vesuvius. What a place to do sweet nothing for a compulsive traveler who has had a hectic lifestyle for what seems like forever and a day!

We have now set intentions for our wellness, UNFORTUNATELY, only after a bout of illness.

Who knew retirement could be so busy? Our schedule is so full we have to say no to many social engagements, and other invitations, "Sorry, we are just too busy," as we peer into our diaries 18 months in advance. At least retirement doesn't feel so strange anymore, the first few months I was totally lost. I awoke at the same time each day, had the same schedule, and then just didn't have to go to work. I have loved my job so much that I thought I'd never retire, but the one-day retirement couldn't come quickly enough, an incident occurred, and as they say, my life flashed before my eyes, and I suddenly wanted to do nothing at all.

Just sit.

Just decompress.

Just smell the air.

Just look out at the views.

Just eat the pizza.

Just sip the vino.

Just finish the day quietly with Torta di Mele, my Nonna's recipe of course, (It's a Apple Pie).

I have not done any of this during my entire working life.

"The stress got to him," a colleague of mine said one day. *What?* I thought, quite offended. I am a quiet, organized and efficient person, empathetic too, and the stress of the job never got to me.

I said to Veridiana one sun-filled morning as we sipped our espresso, stating "I was done."

She dropped her demitasse cup on the porcelain paving and looked at me horrified.

"No, Not us...I'm done with work!" I had to blurt out a laugh, poor Veridiana.

"Let's rebel against a hectic lifestyle and slow down to enjoy life."

Veridiana and I met after my first divorce. We were childhood sweethearts and grew up in the same town; our families know each other very well, and everyone loved each other. We have together honestly lived a blissful life; we have had three children together, and now are what they call 'empty nesters.' Yes, we drink, we eat, we laugh, and have a magnificent life together. She had worked full-time as a professional writer, and with my ALS career, I worked hectic hours, but we always found a way to spend 'some' time doing what we love, but clearly 'not enough' time, we were both sick of rushing everywhere and not enough time for traveling as much as we liked. Then, *THAT* day changed it all for a while.

I was shot in the line of duty

My injury isn't the story I want to tell here, but it is the catalyst for our retirement.

The recovery was long and enduring, Veridiana took great care of me and would wheel me–in the hospital wheelchair– out onto our glorious patio for me to sit in the sun. The scenery was magnificent; snow-capped mountains behind me, and valleys before me. I started to 'notice' my surroundings, 'feel' the breeze, and 'smell' the Lavender in bloom.

I was sweetly doing nothing.

My mind, but I was definitely doing something. A song came on, and I even noticed the words Dolce far Niente, by Mome. It had a little Dicso tone to the song, and I started to bop away in my wheelchair, I found myself repeating it. I peeled a fresh Orange the oils squirting in my face and juice running down my hand, "Dolce farniete, Dolce farniete, Dolce farniete"--bop, bop, bop. Diana (yes, Veridiana) came out and swung me around in the chair, and now we dance in Naples on our new patio, singing these words to each other to the beat of Bella Caio.

Spontaneity also entered our lives at this point.

There is a 72-year-old bookseller, Aziz, located on La Pignasecca in Naples City. It is rather a central thoroughfare, but there is Aziz located in a doorway surrounded by hundreds of books. He sits in the narrow doorway every day; his back sitting on one side of the wall and feet up the wall on the other. He reads and reads and reads for hours each day and chats to the passers-by and those who nod at him. He is always on the same location, he leaves at night and comes back in the morning. His books could be potentially stolen and I asked him one sunny day, and he replied to me that those who can't read don't steal, and those who can aren't thieves. I love his attitude for life.

Whether it be locals sipping their fresh brews at coffee shops, drinking Ale at the foreshore restaurants, or sharing a story walking on the beach, Naples has a common theme— the weather is hot in Summer, streets can be dirty but bustling with life, full of contrasting people and (I've recently discovered) screaming deals on shopping. Yet it has a cloud hanging over its head—Mount Vesuvius and its volcanic eruptions– and burying the beautiful Pompeii.

Diana and I visited the site, Pompeii, and met this amazing woman, Mamia. She changed my view of the world. Venus— the patron of divinity and femininity features significantly in that early society. That day, we learned, that flourishing Pompeii featured that agricultural deity while it's residents basked in the magnificent sun of Italy, as everyone knows, I'm sure, it was buried in the volcanic explosion of A.D 79. Pompeii had an abundance of Olives, fruits, and vegetables and the most wonderful inhabitants. Mamia ran our tour and spoke so highly of the people, and today, the amazing bunch of people who are supporting the history and keeping it alive and relevant—the infinite stories and the infinite nature of keeping this town and its people 'alive', even in the space and time of history. MAGICAL. I LOVE THIS IDEA. Alive–keep the stories alive— no matter what, and everyone lives. That, I feel, is why being involved in this book is so important at this time in my life—and a legacy I can pass on to my family—being published in a book! Everyone in this book and their influential stories, like Dr. Dee, says, their 'little nuggets of gold' and their genius zones, all sharing and speaking highly of others, will remain alive forever—what a legacy to leave.

Noticing, Learning, and then Knowing and Growing:

Nothing refreshes my memory of what I need from the supermarket like coming home from the supermarket!

I never experienced this, either. Diana always did the groceries. It was a new world with different rules in the grocery store — busy Mothers with carts, rushing, elderly with baskets on an adventurous outing, and fit-conscious people who were on a mission to read every word on the labels! I tell you, the Selcar in Mercato is a different world. Next week we are off to Portici, wonder how that will be–life is an adventure. Isn't it interesting, that you bring up your children, live your married life, and work tirelessly in your career, not knowing 'all the different things' that go on in life? Wonder what the people do down in Tore del Greco? Maybe it's time to go there too! Spontaneously! I feel like I've just started to live and see what happening in the world. Maybe it's time for me to 'care' about looking through a different lens. Like Azis and Mamia do?

Enjoyment:

Focus on your wellness brings so many different things to mind.

It eliminates *many* things that don't serve us well; it's time to ditch them. Refrain from cutting out your favorite things, foods included. Use the 90/10 rule. Eat healthy 90% of the time and 10% for enjoyment and bliss, allowing yourself the freedom to enjoy, not just exist. This we now live by, Diana and I are 90/10 people.

Pride:

We are proud to have raised children who can name plants and the herbs, know how to grow foods, know how to cook and cultivate happiness, and celebrate animal life and adventure, not just celebrities, brands, and technology. We are proud of our dedication to our careers and are now proud to be Italians and show our pride for Naples. Everything is interconnected; nothing is separate whereas compassion is everything.

The Infinite:

This continues to Intrigue me. I attend a Gym where I have been doing my rehabilitation work, and now I have joined a team of coss-trainers and their community, there are so many infinite possibilities we can do with our physical body and mind if we 'will' them too. Perform, and imagine into the infinite time and space, and find me in the deepest kind of 'stillness' yet I'm lifting weights, and heavy bars, and rowing and biking with blaring noise and trainers yelling, but I'm at my quietest—all at once. The season of my immense injuries has gone, and now blooming in my own health journey. I sit on our beautiful terrace in Summer, so grateful, the breeze blowing gently and the aromas from my coffee swirling to my nose. Infinite. Thoughts can drown us, thoughts can keep us afloat, and more thoughts can make us fly.

Infinite thoughts.

The infinite is always silent; it only speaks as the finite speaks. Our words are the idle waved caps on a deep ocean that never speaks. We may question the way of science, explain, decide, and discuss, but only in the quiet, and in meditation, and sweetness of sense; The mystery speaks back to us.

Spontaneity, Enjoyment, compassion, and the Infinite; nothing lasts forever. Time is short. This is my message. If you don't set your intentions for your wellness, you will be forced to take time for your illness. People go to work and tragically fail to come home—everyone deserves to come home. To live fast, learn, and grow, we must go slow! Everyone deserves happiness, to experience peace moments, and to be joyous, like Aziz, Mamia, Myself, and Veridiana.

I wish you all too, find a way to be doing Dolce far niente!

I share with you below something that has inspired me for years. Enjoy.

***

L'infinito

Sempre caro mi fu quest'ermo colle,
e questa siepe, che da tanta parte
de l'ultimo orizzonte il guardo esclude.

Ma sedendo e mirando, interminati
spazi di là da quella, e sovrumani
silenzi, e profondissima quiete
io nel pensier mi fingo; ove per poco

il cor non si spaura.
E come il vento
odo stormir tra queste piante, io quello
infinito silenzio a questa voce
vo comparando: e mi sovvien l'eterno,
e le morte stagioni, e la presente
e viva, e il suon di lei.
Così tra questa
immensità s'annega il pensier mio:
e il naufragar m'è dolce in questo mare

***

Infinity

I always have felt a fondness for this lonely hill
and for this hedge, which screens off
such a large part of the furthermost horizon.

But as I sit and gaze, in my thoughts I envisage,
beyond it, boundless space and utter silence
and deepest still, so that it almost makes
my heart take fright.
And as I hear
the rustling of the wind among these plants,
I start comparing that unending silence

with this noise and I am reminded of
eternity, and seasons gone and dead and
of the season now alive and of its sounds.
And so
in this immensity my thoughts sink and drown
and shipwreck feels sweet in this ocean.

(Translation by Phillip Hill)

About the Author

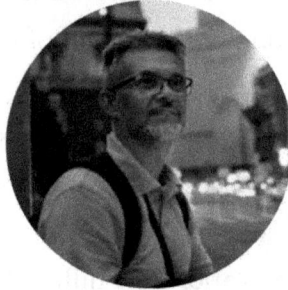

Dr. Lorenzo Bianchi, is the loving husband of Veridiana, now residing in Naples, Italy, blissfully retired from his long-time career of working with the Italian Paramdecis Services as an ALS Physician.

He sits, decompresses, and now lives life more casually than the previous 35 years for 'rush.'

What next for Dr. Lorenzo? Some writing and traveling, more reading, and undoubtedly involvement with the local Naples community and all its colourful vibes.

Email: mynapleslife@gmail.com

-ᴧᴧᴧ→

Suzanna Broughton

Reclaiming Financial Wellness

It is a cold Sunday morning at the tiny home Airbnb with the steep wooden stairs and dim lighting. I am up early, which is unexpected, given how exhausted I am. The kind of exhaustion that sleep will not fix. I told myself that if I woke up, it would be a sign for me to accept the invitation to an online workshop on the subject of my "relationship with time."

So while my partner and dog remained snuggled in their beds, the workshop facilitator started asking questions, and as I answered I realised how much I had lost myself in the preceding months of 2022.

The main thing this workshop reminded me, is that I AM the one making the choices. It was a huge slap in the face to realise I had been exhausting myself and not meeting my own needs.

I did that to me.

But the good news is, since I was the one who did it, I can undo it.

It had been about a year since my partner, Miles, made the decision to leave his job due to new "health" requirements. We could live on one income, and we had significant savings, so this was more opportunity than disaster, however our ongoing savings capacity was all but eliminated.

Home ownership is my big money goal. I am not particularly motivated by money so this goal has a positive effect of keeping me focused on meeting my income goals, which in turn helps me feel a sense of safety and agency. Working towards this goal was my anchor. Not being able to continue working towards the goal was the first domino to fall, and with that my financial wellness began to erode.

Miles and I knew we would be leaving Melbourne Australia for greener pastures. But where to?

A couple of months after Miles left his job he was asked if we could move to New Zealand to help prepare the family farm for sale as Miles' brother received a terminal cancer diagnosis and was unable to continue farming.

Miles was not initially willing to live in New Zealand. He had been there, done that, and he preferred Australia for personal and financial reasons. I had an instant feeling of calm and certainty that we were going. We were needed. This is what life was calling us to do.

After about a hundred more calls, Miles, he who will not be dictated to, eventually *agreed* to the move. I knew he was serious about moving when he sold his cherished MG ZT.

The New Zealand borders were closed, even to Kiwi citizens. Very little went according to plan. Everything from the timing of our move, to where we would live, to what we would specifically be doing once we got there was an exercise in trust and surrender.

The family farm had sold by the time we arrived in New Zealand. We had three weeks to move, give away or burn what remained of 50 years of possessions, farm equipment and the family's rather large car collection. Anything left behind would become property of the new owner who was bulldozing and burning down sheds as soon as we had cleared them out. The pressure was on.

We are so thankful for the help received from generous friends and family, and for their encouragement during those three weeks.

The hardest part for me wasn't leaving my life in Australia, not the expense, not the logistics, not even the culture shock.

The most challenging part was living in the family home and feeling my highly sensitive nervous system bathed in other people's emotions and energies. Every family has their own drama. For best results, give yourself the space you need.

We had not committed to staying in New Zealand; we were here to get a job done, but the job itself was unclear; it started as helping move and mushroomed out as it became apparent that help was needed with legal, accounting, health, and other personal issues.

How can you know when a job is done without clearly defined parameters of what the job is?

Through the transition our finances were precarious. We did not know if we would receive any compensation for our help, or when. I had to completely give up working in my businesses, at least temporarily, as there was no time or energy to dedicate to this. Our expenses were high and unpredictable.

During times of transition, it is imperative that the people going through it give themselves space to work out a plan to meet their needs. They need space to make decisions that best support them.

We were unable to provide ourselves the space we needed. And we did not have the energy or mental clarity to reinforce our will when others overstepped our boundaries. This made it harder for us to meet our basic needs and get jobs done. We felt like we were walking through mud.

I had a genuine desire to do all that I could to support Miles' family during this impossibly hard time. I am also highly empathetic in nature, which causes me to "take on" other people's stuff. I knew logically this was a failed strategy, but logic is usurped when the nervous system is dysregulated. I lost myself trying to help others.

What made it challenging for me to come back to myself was the lack of clarity about the job itself. It is easy to be overwhelmed when there is a lot to do and you do not know where your responsibility begins and ends.

On that cold morning in October, about four months after our hard landing in New Zealand, my nervous system exhaustion was palpable. I wanted to run away from all the problems, from all the pain, and to get myself to a place where I could care for my needs again, rest, and recover.

I was unaware of how small I had made myself in my own life. My brother emailed to share his experience with the 10 year anniversary of my Mother's traumatic death and asking how I was going with it. I realised I had missed the chance to acknowledge this significant passage of time with ritual and celebration. This was another wake-up call. I had lost presence and connection to the things that matter to me.

When the workshop facilitator asked what my current relationship with time is, I answered that I feel busy, like I do not have enough time, and I feel like I do not have the ability to choose what I do with my time.

That last insight was very important.

I had lost sight, not only of my needs, but also of my priorities.

I woke up that morning in more ways than one. I had been asleep to the fact that my relationship with time had gone down the gurgler. I was *feeling* like I did not have the ability to choose. That was not the truth. Feelings are valuable information, but they are not facts.

I consider my relationship with time and my relationship with money to be intricately linked, but this morning I was not thinking about money, or even about time for that matter, I was just feeling a strong pull to "come back to myself".

Coming back to oneself is foundational for creating financial wellness.

I have been consciously crafting my relationship with money for over 10 years and assisting other women to create relationships with money that support them to live with peace, prosperity, and purpose. I am a qualified Certified Financial Planner so planning is entirely my jam. And yet here I was falling into the trap of lack, limitation, and a false belief that I did not have the ability to choose something else, let alone plan for it.

If it can happen to me, it can happen to anyone. Let's normalise needing to review and re-set our financial wellness. There is no shame in admitting the old ways are no longer working and we need a change.

The new rules of financial wellness are not a pre-prescribe formula that everyone must follow. It is about developing the systems and structures that support your financial wellbeing. Sometimes this can mean breaking "old rules". I needed to create new rules because the old rules were not working in my new life.

Following the awareness that I AM the one who is choosing this, things shifted. I was spending far less time lying awake at night, thinking about helping other people with their problems, instead I was lying awake at night thinking about my own problems and how to escape this trap I fell into.

It was clear to me that it was up to us to solve our own problems.

At the time of writing, a year and a half since arriving in New Zealand, we are still wrapping up the job that has taken far longer than anticipated. But now we are a lot clearer where our responsibilities begin and end.

One new rule was to hand back the responsibility, emotions, and burdens that are not mine to carry.

This has freed up so much time and energy for me to focus on my life, my work, my purpose, and supporting Miles while he continues to grow into the man that life is calling him to be. He is such a good man.

This has freed up much needed time and energy to focus on my own financial wellness.

I see three key aspects which encompass the concept of my financial wellness.

- First, there is my *general wellness*, my relationship with time, and my relationship with meeting my own needs. The more I am well in general, the more I am able to focus on activities and decisions that support me in creating financial wellness and prosperity.

- Second, there is the *material financial reality* which is all that is happening with my money in terms of cashflow, wealth, etc. This is what is happening with my money "out there", outside of myself.

- Third, is my *relationship with money*. This is in terms of how my material money reality is impacting me and the meaning I make of it. As well as how I relate to money more generally. It is all the thoughts, beliefs, emotions, perceptions, and stories I have about money. This is what is happening around money inside of myself.

I recognised that my general wellness, my financial reality, and my relationship with money had all drastically changed, in some ways **not** for the better.

Another new rule was to eliminate the outside factors and influences which were not helping and needed to be eliminated.

One of the influences that impacted my relationship with money was issues that arose around intergenerational wealth transfer. I have my own personal experience with this. I have also had many conversations with clients both as a Financial Planner and as a Money Mentor. Potential pitfalls can happen with intergenerational gifts or the promise of gifts in the future:

- When gifts have strings attached, either implied or explicit, this can lead to the receiver feeling controlled, used, and energetically drained.

- Gifts can be demotivating and squash ambition in the receiver.

- Gifts can devalue the receiver's sense of self and the value of their independent lives.

- Promises of gifts that are conditional or do not eventuate can breed entitlement and resentment.

- Issues can arise around perceived inequality among siblings or family members.

It is important for both the givers and the receivers to be aware of these potential pitfalls and more. All of these can impact the receiver's relationship with money, as well as their relationship with the gift givers.

Another new rule that supported me in reclaiming my financial wellness is the awareness that it is me, and only me, who has the power to:

- bring myself back to wellness,

- create positive changes in my material financial reality, and

- create and maintain a functional relationship with money.

Making *external* changes to our financial reality can happen swiftly at times. Other times it can take a while for the pieces to fall into place.

Making *internal* changes to the way we relate to money can happen in a heartbeat. Often, all that is required, is a choice. Once a pattern is seen and recognised, to continue in the same way is a choice.

The following are not rules, but things that supported me to reclaim financial wellness:

- Reflecting on things that I have done well in the past; client reviews and testimonials, past experiences of meeting my goals, even having successfully re-set my financial wellbeing after other transitions.

- Independent paid work which not only provides income but also a sense of accomplishment.

- Valuing my inner work, my inner reality, and my internal direction.

- Focusing on what I am grateful for.

- Being intentional in how I used my time and allowing time for rest.

- Getting involved in communities of people who share my values.

- Finding ways to pay it forward and add value.

- A support system of people to talk to who will really listen, see my value, and reflect back to me the truth in what I am saying.

Some of the above things that helped were really challenging. There were times when I felt really scared, vulnerable, and like I did not matter and nobody cared if I was there or not. On my darkest days I even felt like people would prefer I was not around. I had to keep coming back to sanity and remind myself that although I was feeling that way, feelings are not facts.

Awareness and reflection are essential. I needed to get real with myself about what happened, what role I played, and what role I allowed others to play. I needed to get back to a relationship with money, time and work which is functional and feels positive for me. Talking with Miles for hours, writing hundreds of pages, and crying hundreds of tears has helped me process the experience, move emotional energy, and separate the lessons from the hurricane of confusion.

The last thing I needed was to make myself wrong for looking after my own needs first, and Miles' needs second.

The last thing I needed was to feel guilty as though I did not do enough for others.

It was right for me to take back my place in my own life. That is another new rule.

A decision was made to suck it up. Suck up the financial losses. Suck up any feelings of letdown. Suck it all up and get on with the job of creating true financial wellness, the kind that can only exist when we are honest with ourselves about what we truly want and need.

So I have been doing the hard work. The inner work. The hardest part is not being resentful about how much I have needed to grow to cope and adapt to life. Another new rule is to stop blaming anything outside myself, and instead see the situation for what it truly is; a chance for me to grow.

As a result my capacity to deal with financial uncertainty has expanded, I have put strategies in place so that my finances do not feel so out of control. I have changed the way I relate to financial uncertainty. This is a choice that I was able to make after I woke up and remembered that I AM the one making the choices about how I relate to my finances.

My confidence in my financial future has massively increased, not because I think anyone is coming to save me, but because I know how intensely powerful it truly is to stand in my power and say NO to the things that take me away from myself. I am learning to value my time in new ways.

So many women I have worked with, on the topic of their relationship with money, have said that they want freedom. They do not want to feel like they *have to* do something because of money. They do not want to feel like they *cannot* do something because of money.

My vision for the future, for human beings everywhere, is we continue to break the chains that money, and that people who control money, can bind us up in. That we come to know that true abundance comes from source.

My vision for the future is that money be a tool that we use to empower ourselves. That fear around not having money is dissolved. That we feel connected to source and to all of life, knowing we will always have what we need. That we open our hearts and feel deserving of the many blessings that source provides.

My vision for the future is that we value money enough, just enough, to use it wisely as a powerful tool for crafting beautiful, expansive, and creative lives which bless us and others. That we do not value money too much or put false meanings onto it. That we continue to move away from distorted thinking of lack, limitation, and fear of missing out.

My vision for the future is that we prioritise healing, self-care, meeting our needs, and expressing our creativity over shallow delights that money can buy. That we think deeply about the impact we create in the ways we earn, spend, save, and invest money.

My vision for the future is that we think so highly of ourselves that money can never be used to control us. That we see so clearly our own value that we would never even consider compromising it for money, something that can come and go like a tide.

There is an abundance of money, but there is only one you!

Many blessings for your financial wellness.

About the Author

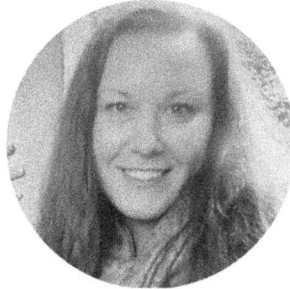

Suzanna Broughton is a former Certified Financial Planner and current Intuitive Financial Healer, Mentor, and Trainer. Feeling chewed up and spat out by the Financial Planning world for thinking differently, Suzanna embarked into self-employment with Her Money Her Purpose.

Using her financial planning training as a base she went on to incorporate unexpected modalities, such as Humanistic Neural Linguistic Psychology and Art of Feminine Presence, into her repertoire to offer women truly unique solutions which take into account the whole woman – not just her money.

She weaves together practical money strategies, with universal principals to creates space for women to transform their relationship with money, and to set up systems and structures to confidently grow their wealth and impact.

Email: Suzanna@hermoneyherpurpose.com
Website: www.hermoneyherpurpose.com
Facebook: www.facebook.com/HerMoneyHerPurpose/

Georgie Grace Carter

There is no force more powerful than a woman determined to rise.

What defines us is how we rise after falling.

My story doesn't begin when I was little or when I was married, it begins the day my abusive marriage ended—abandoned by someone you love is a pain I wish on no one and taking those initial steps alone was terrifying. My heart imploded into a million pieces, and then having to rebuild my life from ashes. Lost and confused with nowhere to call home, I was now homeless and this was my new reality—living on one meal a day with my daughter, our husky Zeva, who I had to rehome. We tried so hard to find somewhere to live. Sounds easy, doesn't it, but in reality, it wasn't. Moments like these are when you find out who your true friends are and if they are willing to help you through these tough times. One person out of all my friends and

55

family put their hand up to take Zeva. This humbled me. Being told by government bodies to put her down as they could only supply my daughter and I accommodation. I would refuse this request until Zeva was safe. I remember telling myself no one is coming to save you. You have to get up and save yourself, so just do it.

Staring into the mirror, I didn't recognise myself. I was 108kg— a shadow of a once bubbly, outgoing, vibrant person before my marriage. What remained of my soul was the smallest ember of light. I had fallen, it was time to rise back up, and little by little I started to reclaim my power. I would wait eight months for a closure that would never come.

So I decided to make one of the hardest decisions, and once it was made, it transformed my life. This decision allowed me to secure a rental property in Mackay. My daughter refers to this as "my saving grace." Looking down at my hand in sheer disbelief that I finally had somewhere safe to call home, a feeling can't be put into words after being abandoned, scared, and homeless. Falling to my knees with tears rolling down my face, I whispered, "We have a place to call home," and I could finally pick up my beloved Zeva. I would now become so driven to embrace life itself. It is a choice to be unstoppable.

This freedom can only be described as a majestic wild horse being set free.

No one could control me and have power over me anymore and I was determined to live the life I was destined for. This is when I decided to make another ripple effect in my journey and join a gym. I became disciplined, driven, and focused on channelling everything I was feeling into that cold bar of steel. It helped lift the enormous weight that I felt on my chest. I know many can relate to this feeling, and the gym saved me in every way a person can be saved. That cold bar of steel doesn't care if you pick it up or not.

There is a moment I reflect on; it was the day I met Shane at the Gym. He would unknowingly restored my faith that decent men still existed.

He said to me: "Keep going and keep focusing on you, don't worry about dating. You're not ready yet."

Slowly, I began to realise he was right. Without his constant reminders, I'm not sure I'd be where I am today. Shane is a true gentleman with a heart of gold, he's passionate about fitness and is highly respected by many. I feel extremely honored to have him a part of my life.

Lachlan would be the other influential male in my life; we shared a passion for pistol shooting and fitness. His encouragement helped me to step out of my comfort zone to achieve goals in both areas I never thought I was capable of. He has always given me his full support in anything I aspire to do.

After graduating year twelve in 1994, I decided to enrol with CQ University and study Certificate III in Fitness after 29 years of being out of school. This became one of the most rewarding experiences of my life. I dedicated myself and never missed one day. Total self-satisfaction hit me when my teachers finally told me that I had graduated, "You are a group instructor GG." I then decided to continue with Certificate IV in Fitness to become a personal trainer. One of my clients recently called me and said, "GG, because of you, I'm a size 16 from being a size 22 for so long. I have never had a personal trainer like you".

When I enrolled in these studies, I was unaware of the challenges that were about to impact me, however, I was so determined and driven. Money was so tight that it became normal to be hungry every day. My most defining moment was having $1.06 in the bank, but I kept finding a way to rise because I hit rock bottom, which became the solid foundation for rebuilding my life. I had no other option but to sell my personal items to buy food and fuel, and to continue my studies. Often feeling disheartened by the choices I had to face, my daughter then told me, "Mum, I have never met anyone like you, you always seem to find a way around an impossible situation. You are like a Phoenix rising from the ashes".

Soon after graduation, I was encouraged to run the CQUniversity boot camp for staff and students on campus. This became a very proud moment and a milestone of my success. I have been told, "Wow, you have honestly turned your trauma into triumph, and you haven't realised it."

The Phoenix Rising - unstoppable!

I want to take this opportunity to thank the teachers who have supported and guided me through all my studies with CQU. Nina, Russel, Ashleigh, and Linda— have reshaped and transformed me into who I am today. I honestly believe I would not be the person I am today without all of them.

Through life we have a memorable defining moment—an epiphany, and mine occurred while doing a business assessment. We were given questions that would make us look deeper into our "WHY". Who do you want your clients to be? What would you call your business? These questions would unknowingly be the key to a door that was about to swing wide open. My teachers helped me realise "You are not defined by what happened to you".

"Who are you, GG "? With the sudden realisation that I was tenacious and genuine and not defined by what I went through. This was the moment I knew what my business name would be called, it would be "Fire and Grace Fitness." This is who I am. "Fire in my soul and Grace in my heart."

The Phoenix Rising- Unstoppable- Fire and Grace.

After achieving a 35 kg weight loss in 18 months, I aspire to compete in a range of fitness competitions in 2026. I have no glass ceiling to what I want to achieve; I have the dedication and discipline to make this a reality. Limitless is the only word that comes to mind. You can support me or get right out of the way because everything in my life has prepared me for this inevitable moment.

"You will see many changes in her, but the most beautiful is the change in her eyes: they are much clearer, wiser, penetrating, and compassionate."

Working at PCYC as a group and personal trainer has brought me to my next milestone. There is a statewide program called "Ruby"(Rise Up Be Yourself) that I would love to be a part of. Transforming someone into a stronger, healthier version of themselves is the most rewarding experience. You share that journey, building a stronger mind and body to form a powerful transformation. Now she flies.....

The Phoenix Rising - Unstoppable - Fire and Grace - Flying Limitlessly!

If you've ever experienced a rush of euphoria after an evening of dancing, you would know firsthand that dancing is good for the soul. I have read studies that have shown dancing boosts mental health and keeps the brain healthy. This is where my circle of friends and I meet—on the dance floor!

So I ask you, my dear readers, "What sets your soul on fire?"

If you've not found it or lost it, stay with me for this journey, for grapes must be crushed to create wine, diamonds are made under great pressure, and seeds grow in deep darkness.

So whenever you feel crushed, under immense pressure, or trapped in the darkness, know that you are in a powerful process of growth and transformation. This analogy has helped me over the years. Never allow anyone to dictate that you can not make a change. Only you have the power to be part of a positive ripple effect. At this very moment, you are capable of making an extraordinary difference in the world. Even a simple small deed can make a profound impact on the life of another, so create a ripple that will turn into a wave. I am now focused on living my most authentic life—happier, smarter, and working hard to live unapologetically doing what I love.

The Shift

There are certain people who will enter your life who will enrich your journey in ways you never believed possible. I was told when I was very little, "If you can count on one hand your genuine friends, you are very rich." How true this statement was. Today, I can say I am rich with the circle of friends that stand beside me.

When I started to rebuild my life, I was driven to achieve

everything I had ever wanted to aspire to. I had always wanted to do competition pistol shooting, so one day I decided to walk into the local gun shop. That is when I met Laura. She supported and guided my journey, and before long, we became close friends. It never crossed my mind that she actually owned the shop until the boys at the range told me. She made me realise I was a strong, independent woman who was whole on my own. She has nurtured me through all the obstacles I have faced. I couldn't imagine my life without Laura not to mention the memes she sends to keep me in line.

The Lord also placed another special woman into my life at a networking meeting for Fire and Grace. This was when I met Nathenea— we have so many beliefs, interests, and goals in common. We meet regularly for dinner and dancing, which would become the highlight at the end of our busy week. One night, Nathenea introduced me to Grace, an extraordinary singer of a local band—G-Force—her voice is a true gift from God, as is her beautiful soul. We became good friends and then Grace welcomed me into her family for Christmas 2023. Our sisterhood group consisted of so many beautiful ladies: Sharon, Melay, Margaret, NuRr, and Venus—all understanding who I am and to be my authentic self—Strong independent, and driven. Whether on the dance floor or at McDonald's at 3 am laughing about the night we just had, we are the friends that became family—empowering and supporting each other to rise together. There is a verse in the Bible from Thessalonians 5:11 that says,

"Therefore encourage one another and build one another up." I love that.

Nathenea asked me to accompany her to church one Saturday, and I accepted immediately. I can only describe the feeling like I was finally home. I felt so loved amongst so many welcoming arms. I had missed this for so long. It is easy to get lost and lose our way, but from time to time I would pray for guidance and I believe my prayers were finally answered. This was a moment I'll never forget, I knew exactly who I was and who I was meant to be. That is a very powerful place to be. I no longer seek validation from anyone. I'm just living my life in my own lane and working on my life goals.

As I rediscovered who I was, I began to read a book that truly impacted my life, The Complete Book of Rules by Ellen Fein and Sherrie Schneider— insight to capture the heart of Mr Right. It changed my life, and I suggest you go out and find the book. I highly encourage every woman to read it.

When someone comes out of a toxic relationship, we are foreign to what normal love is. We have been conditioned and have to unlearn everything we were told. This book explained all the challenges that I have faced. Money was extremely tight; I often daydreamed about being able to afford a holiday, having a break, or even getting dressed up for an event. However I knew I could only barely afford enough food. These tough times have made me appreciate everything I have in life. Some nights, I would pray for the moment to feel pretty again.

This is when a friend placed her ticket to an event called 'Banquet En Blanc' - a white party. Leanne from Silk Laser Clinic posted on Facebook, "Who is doing it tough and would like a free ticket to this event"? At first, I hoped it went to someone who would really appreciate it and I kept scrolling on. Then the post came up again in my news feed, and I then reached out to her and said that life has been a little hard and I'd love to go. She responded, "It's all yours, do you have an outfit to wear?". I cried in disbelief it was actually mine—I was overwhelmed by her generosity, and kindness. Less than twenty-four hours before this event, I became nervous. I was amongst four hundred strangers was so empowering to only say" Hi, my name is Georgie Grace." That was it. The first girl I introduced myself to was Jo, and on this mysterious trip, saying to her, "I'm here alone." Jo replied, " Man, you got some balls turning up to an event on your own, wow." I laughed and said, "I embrace all life has to offer".

You have friends for a reason, friends for a season, and friends for a lifetime. Never forget who has impacted your life.

The Unstoppable Me

I have become that woman determined to rise and is truly unstoppable. Looking at my reflection in 2024, I stand independent, strong, and determined to live the life I've always deserved.

To live by one's passion is to live your most authentic life, Pistol shooting and Photography are mine. Yes, you heard right, my other favorite pastime is pistol shooting. Why not?

Many people fear this sport and say they couldn't imagine doing it, but that is exactly what limits your imagination, this is when you give it a go. I embrace life and enjoy the thrill of the competition to become better than I was yesterday. A comfort zone is a beautiful place, but nothing ever grows there. Like I said before, I will not limit myself to a glass ceiling at anything I want to achieve now. We are limited only by our own minds.

My camera is this intriguing device that captures the world the way I see it.

As a child, I never put it down. No two photographers will ever take the same photo, we all have a unique fingerprint on how and what we see. That's what makes it so incredible. We are all very unique in what we do. A photograph, with one single click, is then frozen at that precise moment, only capable of returning back to that time through that photograph. The picture you hold on that photographic paper of your loved one, a pet that may have passed, or an event that you wish you could relive. All your senses overwhelm you at once looking at this picture, you have been taken back to that exact moment again. That is the most rewarding ability you can hand someone. Embracing nature and photographing wildlife is my happy place. I have showcased my wildlife photography in competitions that led me to win first place and printed in outback calendars for numerous years.

I also have a strong passion for wellness, natural medicine, and herbs.

As a child, I was constantly sick, and on a regular basis, I had to see a doctor. Having asthma from an early age was only the beginning. If I got sick, it normally led to Bronchitis, and in one case, it led to me being put into the hospital with severe Pneumonia. Losing my Mum to Lung Cancer was the moment my hands felt completely tied, I felt paralyzed by the fact I couldn't help her. This was my turning point, and embarked on research with natural medicine. Then I met Katrina, owner of 'The Health Nut' health food shop. Not only a close friend but also she's like my second Mum and she asked if I wanted to work with her at her shop. The answer was a big HELL YEAH!

Knowledge is power, and I would stop at nothing to learn more. Traveling to Brisbane to attend Nutrition summits and truly embrace myself in what I love. All things related to natural health, studying books, listening to podcasts - all this has inspired me to go further. and I have developed my own rules around health and wellness that I want to follow with F.L.Y: FIRST LOVE YOURSELF.

Today is also another triumphant day—I finally obtained a four-bedroom house with a two-bay garage. I have waited three painful years for this moment, and as I was given the keys to this property, another step from trauma to triumph. Walking into such a massive place after living so humbly for years is a feeling you can't describe. I am so grateful for what I have and feel blessed in many ways. It still overwhelms me that this place is mine. I have a photography room and a place where I can even edit my photos. Thank You God.

Fire and Grace has organically attracted a like-minded community and I have created a support group to help encourage my clients' journey. I want to make a *real* difference in the community and have a positive impact on the lives of many. I have received so much support from the community and encouragement. Not to mention a statewide program I am destined to be part of shortly. I want Fire and Grace to be a legacy. I will do everything in my power to make this a reality. I am whole, I do not need the validation of others to love myself, I know exactly who I am and I stand strong. A group I have worked with told me:

"Georgie-Grace, you are one of the strongest, bravest authentic women that I've come across, you give me goosebumps about what you will achieve next".

I am truly blessed to have support from all my friends and the local businesses in my community.

Everything I have gone through has brought me to the remarkable woman who stands before you. If you didn't go through it, you wouldn't be YOU! Who would I be if I hadn't gone through it all? My exterior is strong, and my interior is even stronger with a mindset determined to make a massive impact on changing how fitness is seen— It has to hurt you.

You need to feel the pain to get the reward or you don't appreciate the destination. What defines you is how well you rise after falling. My hand will be there if you reach out. I'd love to connect with you and discuss your new transformation further.

Unleash the FIRE in your soul, and GRACE within your heart and rise to become the best version of yourself. There is no force more powerful than a woman determined to rise.

Georgie Grace Carter. xo

About the Author

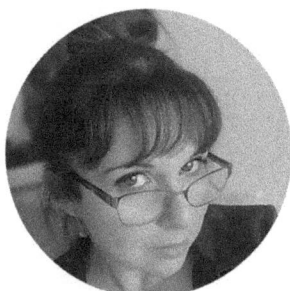

Georgie Grace Carter is a creative genius, tenacious and genuine, a true transformational woman, and assists others in being their best selves. Within her business—Fire and Gace Fitness—she is a qualified Personal Trainer and Group Fitness Instructor who is involved in many community programs.

In her personal time you may find her unwinding at the beach— a true "Sunshine and saltwater" gal, adoring the seashells and walking in her bikini as the Sun goes down.

This is who Georgie-Grace truly is, so alive and unapologetically passionate — wandering barefoot in search of a piece of driftwood to create artwork with in the sand, drawings that would later be erased by the saltwater tide.

Email: fire.grace.fitness@gmail.com
Facebook: https://www.facebook.com/fireandgracefitness11
Instagram: fire_and_grace_fitness

-∿∿>

Jason Chapman

'No one owes you anything.' ~ Jason Chapman

I wake up in a sweat, the bed sheets are drenched, and I cannot get the image out of my mind. A reoccurring dream plagues me—A young boy looks out the back window of a car while it drives away down the country road, looking at that soon-to-disappear woman just standing there on the side-flank in tears. The boy's hot hand quickly pressed against the rear glass like a scene from the Titanic. The little boy was me, the woman was my Mother, and I grew up in a split family.

I was drenched in sweat daily, not from the recurring dream from my past, but from the symptoms and diagnosis of Hodgkins' Lymphoma— I was 17 years old when I was diagnosed. It came as a lightning bolt out of nowhere, and my entire world changed at that moment, sitting in the doctor's office, numb. Now, it's ten years on. I'm a survivor, thriving surrounded by an immense supportive network and fully embracing the present moment. Letting go often starts with being fully present, practicing mindfulness, and immersing myself in the current moments. Having your attention forced to focus on the present, you naturally release a grip on the past and worries of the future, not to say fear doesn't rise, for it does regularly, and sometimes, on some days, I feel am plagued by fear too, yet being present allows you to experience life as it unfolds, unburdened by the unnecessary baggage.

I sit in a dark cupboard amongst the clothes, holding a large box of assorted pills.

Time stands still. My mind tells me 'to take them all,' hell, 'Just do it,'. My other inner voice says, 'Reach out for help, talk to someone.'

I frantically call many different help and crisis line numbers, the counselors on the other end just listening to my erratic sobs, all resulting in no help at all–to my surprise. The last report hit me — call the hospital ward I had been staying in for my treatment and, by chance, got one of my amazing nurses. She expressed her fond memory of me, and we chatted for what felt like hours (I'm sure it wasn't, but time was stagnant at that moment).

Thank the Universe of Nurses, our Earth Angels!

I know I am here today due to the support of others, so now this has elevated my insane need and desire to be there for others, too, when needed, especially those experiencing a journey that is unexplainable, a journey that is the most difficult, a journey that feels like it will never end.

In times of need, REAL NEED, who answers calls?

Who is ever there for others? Who feels the love behind others' needs? Who listens to someone sobbing so hard that they are snorting and not even getting a word out?

Delta Goodram, Australian Musician, Songwriter, Actress, TV personality, and HL survivor and warrior, once said, "Anybody who has gone through a life-changing experience will tell you there is a different understanding of what is real and what is important, and when you are going through different moments, you can reflect and go, ' I have been through worse.'"

To be honest, she has unofficially been my mentor throughout my journey, and one day, I dream of thanking her in person, informing her of the inspiration by proxy in my own Hodgkin's journey. When I felt weak and broken or like giving up, I would look at her on YouTube, listen to her music and really deeply feel her words, and say, "WOW- look at her now." I knew I had this in the bag. I watched all that she publicly had to offer; I inhaled it all as inspiration. I imagine feeling elated if she ever picked up a copy of this book and saw my story and how she impacted my life…hope that happens!

I am currently living a dream.

My husband and I hold an itinerant vibe; we love change, moving around our amazing country, Australia, and experiencing different things—WE LIVE AND LOVE LIFE!

He is the most amazing person in my life; the love, the support, the reciprocated empathetic ear, my emotional everything—and when my fear surfaces, and he is my calm, our connection is blissful…and we are creating magic in our lives— we even now have a growing investment portfolio! WINNING!

It became clear to me why the universe had allowed me to do what I did – it was because it led me to meet the love of my life, now my husband. No more 'Back on Tinder' moments where I would swipe through profiles, hoping to find a connection. From that day forward, we never left each other's side, and our connection grew stronger with time. We now choose to live in North Queensland, living our best life, and I'm about to embark on an Authorship experience and one day have a hobby farm.

My parents still heavily feature in our lives too. At the beginning of my chemo sessions, both my Mum and Dad would accompany me for support. It meant a lot to have them by my side, especially considering that I was the youngest patient receiving treatment at the hospital during that time. (However, our collective presence was short-lived when someone complained about me having two people with me instead of adhering to the hospital's rule of only one person being allowed during treatment.)

It all started, and this one morning was etched in my mind: I woke up to excruciating pain in my arm.

It felt like someone had been sitting on it, and the pins and needles sensation was unbearable. Despite the limited mobility, I still went to work. But halfway through the day, the pain became too much to bear, and I had no choice but to rush to the hospital. Upon undergoing an ultrasound, it was revealed that I had developed a blood clot in my arm.

The agony I experienced in my arm over the following days was the most intense pain I had ever felt.

It served as a stark reminder of the challenges and complications during my chemotherapy treatment; I vividly recall my stubbornness from the very beginning. The doctors had suggested that I have a PIC line (a catheter inserted through a peripheral vein in the arm) inserted into my arm to make the chemo process easier on my veins, as the treatment can be quite harsh on them. However, as a stubborn 17-year-old, I was resistant to the idea. If I had the PIC line, I wouldn't have a blood clot. After each chemo session, the nurses faced increasing difficulty finding accessible veins for the treatment. Eventually, they reached a point where they couldn't access my veins anymore. It was during one particular chemo session, with my best friend Katie by my side that the nurses attempted four times to insert the needle until it became clear that I had no choice but to get a PIC line. Overwhelmed, I covered my face with my hood, curled up into a ball, and cried for a good 10 minutes on the chemo chair, ending up wishing I had done it from the start. The absence of needle pain during the chemo sessions made the whole experience much more bearable. Looking back, I regret my stubbornness and wish I had been more open to the idea earlier.

New Rule of Wellness: Let go of stubbornness!

One aspect of my treatment that I found incredibly challenging was its impact on my appearance. As a 17-year-old who took pride in my appearance, I loved my hair and enjoyed applying makeup daily. I didn't care about the judgmental looks I received because what mattered most to me was feeling good about myself. However, when treatment began, I noticed my hair thinning out. I vividly remember driving home from chemo, running my fingers through my hair, and discovering a ball of hair in my hands. It was devastating. Not only was I losing my hair, but the steroids I was taking also caused rapid weight gain. I ended up gaining around 30 kilograms in total. The sudden growth caused stretch marks to appear, and I would sit in front of the mirror, shocked and in tears, unable to recognize myself.

It was a heartbreaking experience.

Another New Rule of Wellness: Do what it takes to make yourself feel good, no matter the opinions of others!

I also hold a vivid memory of my first experience with chemotherapy. I recall walking to the toilet, pushing along my IV trolley that was connected to the bags of chemo. As I went to urinate, I was taken aback when I saw that my urine was a bright red color. Panic rushed over me, and I immediately thought that I was dying. With tears streaming down my face, I hurried back to the chemo room and approached the nurse, expressing my fear and belief that the worst was happening to me. The nurse kindly tried to comfort me, explaining that the red color was simply a result of the chemo I was receiving. Specifically, the chemo I had, known as ABVD, contained the infamous "red devil" component—Red Devil indeed!

After undergoing chemo, I experienced intense sickness for three days. During this time, I had a strong aversion to any light in the room. All I desired was a completely dark environment where I could find solace and sleep. I spent those three days mostly sleeping, trying to find relief from the discomfort. However, my sleep was often interrupted by severe heart palpitations, causing anxiety and fear to consume me. There were moments when I would wake up believing that my heart might stop beating and that I wouldn't wake up again. The constant worry and uncertainty added to the already challenging experience. Sometimes, even today, I have thoughts of life and death and how long I'm going to live—I guess none of us know.

In the chemo room, there were four chairs positioned to face each other. This arrangement meant that during each chemo session, I would sit across from a random person receiving treatment. Surprisingly, this setup was beneficial as it encouraged conversation and interaction.

During my chemo sessions, I had the opportunity to meet many individuals going through similar experiences. We would exchange tips and share treats, discussing helpful foods or random items that brought comfort during treatment. One particular older lady I met was exceptionally kind and compassionate. We would engage in conversation for the entire six hours of our sessions. We would discuss our treatments and share what had effectively alleviated our symptoms. To my delight, on one occasion, when I arrived for chemo, I discovered that the kind lady had left me a heartfelt card along with some beautiful flowers to give to me. This gesture brought me immense joy and gratitude. It was a touching reminder of the connections and support that can form during such challenging times.

My hematologist is an incredible woman.

I vividly recall our first meeting. She glanced at me as I walked into her office, "Why the heck are you here? You're way too young!" My Mum and I exchanged glances, and we couldn't help but burst into laughter. At that moment, I knew she was the doctor I needed, someone who not only possessed exceptional medical expertise but also felt like a friend. I felt comfortable asking her any question, no matter how difficult or uncomfortable the topic was. She was genuine, down-to-earth, and had a great sense of humor. The best part was that she had a knack for making me laugh, even during those serious discussions. Having a doctor like her was a blessing, as she provided top-notch medical care and genuine human connection and support.

Once again, my stubborn nature emerged during my chemotherapy journey.

The internal battles I fought daily were overwhelming. The constant conflict within myself was unimaginable. However, I persevered and pushed through, determined to maintain a sense of normalcy. I've always had a block talking about myself; I really enjoy hearing about other people's lives and life adventures and bringing this back to my writing now, I feel a sense of sharing my life and adventures, and it's my time to share my story, the time is right to share.

Every day, I think about what kind of hobby I would love to have and what else I can do that enriches me. A way to be fully present, practice my mindfulness in new, fun ways, and immerse myself in the current moments. I don't have a favorite book as an adult, but as a child, I used to love "The Faraway Tree" novel series. Enid Blyton had me on many journeys through enchanted woods with Fairy-Folk and colourful characters like Moon-Face and Saucepan-Man sliding through magical slip-and-slides curling inside the trunk of a huge special tree—The Faraway Tree. I would love to design and make my clothes. My Mother got me a sewing machine for Christmas, but it's in Adelaide, so I have to find a way to get it.

I would also love to have my hobby farm or learn a new random skill— like building something. But for right now, my favorite thing would be just lounging in a swimming pool, gazing up at the sky, and listening to all the different birds. As I grew up in South Australia, the birds and bugs all sounded different, and now I am enjoying not being cold all the time!

What would I do if I had all the time and money— I would have a small hobby farm, similar to a wildlife park, where visitors Make donations. These donations would go towards the Redkite Foundation, as they had helped my Mum a lot when we needed them my Mum had to put a hold on her mortgage when I was sick, but other bills didn't stop coming in, and Redkite was their Redkite helped pay for Mums electricity bills water bills and all those bills when she wasn't making an income because she was looking after me and Redkite was actually who paid for me to get my first truck license, my MR. I'm still so grateful for that and won't be fulfilled until I give that money back so they can help other people in need. They are a great foundation, and I've decided the profits I make from this book can go towards them.

I've always had a love for the land and animals.

As a child, I had a massive chicken coop. We had about 30 chickens. At one point, I had about 72 racing pigeons/homing pigeons. I had five Peking ducks and a cage full of budgies, and the first thing I think about when asked that question is my favorite thing: sitting in the middle of the cage and watching all the animals doing their own little thing every morning. When at Dad's house, I would wake up, and that was the first thing I did - went straight to the chicken cage and sat there. It didn't matter if it was 42° outside; I would be in the tin shed making sure they were all okay. My brother used to always hang out at the neighbor's house, and they used to go fishing and crabbing all the time. I didn't enjoy hanging out with them, but they were the only option for company. I remember the neighbor approaching me once and inviting me to join them. His wife had scolded him for never including me in their activities. but I told him, "All good, I'm happy doing my own thing."

I remember when I finally made friends with one kid there. I enjoyed his company, which is rare, and we got along. He watched a movie, and I showed him my animals. It was great to have someone else interested in my animals finally. Then he left after an hour or two.

I went to grab my headphones, wanting to go for a walk along the beach, listening to music and watching the sunset. It's also one of my favorite things. And they were gone, looking everywhere for them. It came to my mind that he may have taken them, so I went over there and went to the front door like a peeping Tom, looking through the window of the front of the house. I saw him sitting on the couch with them. How I knew they were them they were stained with pen as a pen leaked through my pants the other week. So I went and got my dad and told him, thankfully, I got them back.

It's my dream to own my own little hobby farm one day at the heart is a beautiful garden that attracts the native fauna. I will enjoy being fully present, practicing mindfulness, and immersing myself in the current moments.

Another memory that made me have the focus and care I do today is, During that time, my friend invited me to the year 12 formal, and I was grateful for the opportunity to still have that experience. However, on that night, I could hear people whispering about me, saying things like, "That's the guy with cancer." Even the teachers approached me to ask how I was doing, which I guess I should have expected, but at the same time was hoping no one knew. For a few years, if I was introduced to someone around my age and they seemed to know me, they would refer to me as "the guy that had cancer."

Reach out if you need support, to chat, or to feel love surrounds you. I want you to know you're growing into a beautiful garden in my heart. Help is available–speak, for emotional support is most valuable. Although I deeply feel that No one owes you anything, it's comforting to know that other people are out there, well here, that both care deeply and love deeply.

Life is a journey I don't have a map for. I believe the impossible is possible to overcome, believing in miracles born from love in everyone.

About the Author

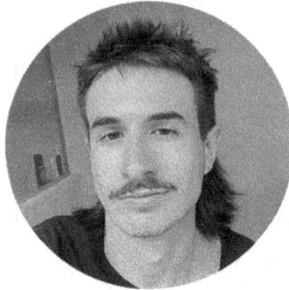

Jason is transforming his life and assisting others organically as it unfolds; his journey is nothing short of amazing. From treatment to thriving, he knows being there with a loving heart for others on their journey is lifesaving.

Suppose he is not down the duck park feeding his feathered friends with his $18/a bag of chicken food (not bread—specifically white bread) or sitting by the Airport watching the planes come and go. In that case, you will find him scooting around with his little UberEats bag, not for the money, but for the love of social interaction, the service, and the gratitude that shows up in the smiles of others. Each morning when he feels he needs an extra energy boost, he dons his 'Luky-Duck' pearlescent earrings and slays-the-day—-on other days, his choice is his Kangaroo earrings to hop into the day with a positive attitude!

Email: jason_chapman51@ymail.com
Facebook: www.facebook.com/jason.chapman.11
Instagram: jasonjchapman

-Ⱳ⟶

Stephanie Christine

I would never have thought that the topic of energies, frequencies, greatness, and toxins would captivate me so much, and sitting here typing and writing, peering into my screen as if looking out of my small inner world into the great expanse of the infinite universe. But questions and frequencies occupy my head space: Who am I? What got me there? What is life about? Amongst all of it, it took me quite some time to understand that life is meant to be this way. That everything that is happening is happening for you, not to you. Life is creating opportunities and space for growth. What aspects of my life led me here and writing... Well, I can only connect the dots backward. Life has always been meant to be this way.

For me, and many globally, in March 2020, humanity seemed to have come to a standstill — life in standby mode. Just a month earlier, in February, the decision to embark on a new business adventure was made. And I am telling you, the journey to this decision was long and bumpy. Doubts were a daily companion. Would I even be up to it? But the decision was made, and between all the doubt, there was excitement, anticipation, and a new thirst for adventure. And suddenly, just a few weeks later, life seemed to come to a standstill. Welcome again: Fear, worry and doubt. But I walked the walk; there was no way to go back. And the extent of the impact it would have on me, my life, and the lives of thousands of people was unforeseeable. This time, they have opened up entirely new perspectives and insights. Encounters, experiences, and emotions gradually connected all the dots. Slowly, they began to make sense, and the sense that this was precisely what had to happen became clear.

All the work, experiences, encounters, and emotions made me realize the following and led to this beautiful encounter that I have the opportunity to write about here:

Your BODY is a beautiful ensemble of a spiritual, emotional, mental, and physical body. Everything is connected. And your body is the instrument for creating your life. Everything is energy that vibrates at a particular frequency. And your body is such a fine vessel to transmute the energy. It carries infinite wisdom and potential. Potential that you may not even be aware of. As humans, it is our purpose and responsibility to unveil as much of this potential and wisdom as possible, to master the multilayer

of our body, to uncover the greatness, and to stand up as sovereign beings.

I invite you on a journey: Visualize a seed, a beautiful apple seed! Imagine this tiny seed being planted. It requires water, the warmth and the light of the sun, good nutritious soil, and time. It just evolves. Its innate intelligence turns the tiny seed into a healthy apple tree with delicious and nutritious fruit. It's all there. Knowing and perfection rest in the seed. There is just as much knowing and intelligence in us humans. This inner wisdom enables us to grow, evolve, recover, and regenerate.

Let's dive into the realm of energy. And I don't mean in the sense of putting the plug into the socket. Imagine everything surrounding us is energy, you are energy. As Einstein said, "Everything is energy, and that's all there is to it." Einstein as well – „Energy cannot be created or destroyed, it can only be changed from one form to another." Tapping into this understanding is huge because **your body is the instrument to create your life. Your body is this fine vessel that transforms energy into physical matter.**

The soil on which your fruits grow, the fruits of life. It is greatness; it is perfection. You are greatness! You are perfect!

But who am I to say this?

My life wasn't always backed up with greatness and sovereignty. I grew up pretty normal. Born at the end of the 70s on the edge of Berlin, in the former eastern part of Germany. It was a time when the Cold War was still in full bloom, and the Iron Curtain was more than upright and impenetrable. This time and this part of the world were characterized by conformity: Full employment for men and women, a „flourishing modern healthcare system" with immunization of society through vaccines and antibiotics. Childcare from a very early age onwards was standard. Some energies awakened the ambition to be higher, faster, stronger, and better but not to step out of line. This way, conformity and a prevailing political value system could be maintained. In contrast, I saw that family and community cohesion were present and essential qualifications.

I was performing averagely at school, active in sports, and talented. Later on, I became aware that I carried a lot of fear around making mistakes and not conforming. I'm glad I grew up in a historically impressive time and area. I was 12 when the Berlin Wall came down, and life, people, and the view of life, or rather the possibilities of it, changed dramatically. My family was very close-knit, but I was drawn out into the world... There was an inner urge to go out and get to know my own world.

Other important milestones were a high school year abroad and studying on the other side of Germany. Life happens for you... not to you. Every experience, no matter how uncomfortable it may be, is meant to happen. They are opportunities to grow and to evolve. Inside, the seed was clearly recognizable. I was not made for conformity.

There weren't the highly fascinating adventures that had a formative influence on my life. Still, all in all, it was a multitude of little things that allowed me to have precisely those experiences that are so significant for my current perspective. As mentioned, you can only connect the dots looking backward. But who am I? What did me get there? Well, it took me quite some time to understand that life is meant to be this way. That everything that is happening is happening for you, not to you.

Isn't life amazing where it takes you? A couple of micro-experiences, superficially nothing special at all, led me to Austria and giving birth to the two most beautiful and influential teachers in my life, my two boys, who are, at the time of writing this, 14 and 17 years of age. Motherhood is an adventure on its own, an adventure we can talk about over a cup of coffee, but raising and taking over responsibility of these two beautiful humans created situations, that led to a series of decisions; it has introduced me to people who have tremendously impacted my life. But it also changed my perspective on life many times. It was overwhelming to a certain degree, but it was so valuable at the same time. For me, it was an adventure of breaking out of the old common ways of thinking, acting, and behaving. Did I take the smooth and easy way? Is there even a smooth and easy way? From my perspective - No way! Learning and changing are rarely smooth and easy. But it's worth it.

After the discovery of different alternative approaches to health and well-being and more and more trust in the natural powers of our own bodies, the path to body therapy opened up. There was still a missing piece that wanted to be discovered. The journey into energetics had begun with the

adventure of Shiatsu. From the intention to learn a craft, something much greater emerged. The first touches on the fact that energies flow within us, that these can be blocked and have a corresponding effect on our well-being — consciously or unconsciously.

This truly has been the time to break out of conformity and go into critical thinking. Just like every mom, I wanted the best for my boys, and I did have the luxury of meeting amazing people during pregnancy and during the time when my boys were little. It led me to a holistic approach to seeing health and taking care of it — This process of raising two! This journey became an impactful personal experience.

Out of the urge to be truly independent, a new search began... A search for alternatives to the classic economic systems, a search for oneself. The call for freedom grew louder and louder

— freedom in development and a life outside the classic systems that made me feel ill. And then I was faced with it — decisions again. Even if the intention was good, the next step was not without hurt and pain — the choice of a new life and a new partnership. Digesting and processing this step took time. Time for reorientation, growth, and processing.

There it was — finally breaking out of my skin, breaking free from conforming, and genuinely discovering my personal truth and the new rule of wellness. You can only connect the dots backward — Life has always been meant to be this way. My journey took me to Salzburg, Austria, in March 2019. The venue was a well-known coffee house chain, where the first seeds for a new business adventure were planted, which eventually started to really grow almost a year later before humanity was sent into standby mode a month later.

The Moment my life changed was within the space of my New Business Opportunity and my innate action — purely out of trust, and the world suddenly opened up in a whole new light. There was doubt and insecurity. There were efforts to revive my previous business. Nevertheless, the magic was gone, though the (perceived) responsibility remained. I also knew that I did not ever want to return to living an ordinary life that fits into a 9-5 box or requires a stationary office building. There was this urge for adventure and growth. Of course, I was aware of my responsibility towards my kids, but it was challenging to agree to a traditional model of life. If you truly want something and make a decision about it, it will fall into place eventually.

A real test of confidence and conviction. Trust in the unseen.

The decision was made. Society in standby mode - What a crazy time that brought so many secrets to the surface. It gave me a whole new perspective on life. At first, I just sat there shaking my head and couldn't believe it. Later, the responsibilities and possibilities became apparent. The dots connected.

The trust has paid off; my North Star was unveiled. I realized that I was holding something unique in my hands — a solution, a paradigm shift.

My discovery: We all have a perfect inner piece that carries infinite wisdom. We are sovereign beings but numbed by life; our perception is limited. The pineal gland is switched off. There are ways and possibilities to reactivate all of this. But it is up to us. We can step back into our sovereignty and *be* ourselves.

But why is it so challenging to tap into this infinite wisdom, into sovereignty, into peak performance? Why do people get highly motivated,   inspired, and easily brought back to their environment where everything seems lost? We say this is human; this is the human mind. And yes, to a large degree, this is true for sure, but are you aware that exposure to toxins and heavy metals from the environment has an unfavorable effect on people's brains and overall performance?

People are burdened with toxins and heavy metals from the environment, as well as from their own lifestyle, which has a negative impact on their health, emotions, and performance. No one would argue that our body holds miracles within — But do we really know? Do we really understand, and do we treat it this way?

Journalist Sydney J. Harris stated:

> "Ninety percent of the world's woe comes from people not knowing themselves, their abilities, their frailties, and even their real virtues. Most of us go almost all the way through life as complete strangers to ourselves."

Most humans are not aware. Hardly anyone is performing at their highest level. A lot of negativity, illness, depression, and anxiety characterize today's world. People are getting sicker and sicker and are facing increasing health and life challenges.

Why is no one asking?

As humans, we are multilayer beings. We have a physical body, a mental body, an emotional body, and a spiritual body. Everything is interconnected; nothing is separate. And it is precisely in this finely networked space that so much potential lies that we humans have yet to tap into. And when all the elements of our being are optimally connected, in balance and in communication, when everything is integrated with and into each other, then all this potential can be released.

We are nature. We are a divine design.

Transmuting energies: Everything is energy. Thoughts are energy. Energy can not be created or destroyed. It can only be transmuted. That's a law. And our body, as a divine composition of the physical, mental, emotional, and spiritual, is the vessel to transmute energies. It is the instrument to create life by law. This state of unity allows us to perform in the highest possible way. It is pure greatness.

We are a masterpiece with abilities and skills to
self-regulate and regenerate.

We live in natural relationships, connections, and dependencies with our environment, nature, and others. And that's precisely what is becoming increasingly toxic, pushing all those fine connections out of balance, allowing people to operate only at a fraction of their potential. Environmental toxins like aluminum, mercury, cadmium, glyphosate, etc.,   cause imbalance and isolation — isolation on the cellular level as well as amongst humans and nature. As within so without. Imbalance and isolation are causing illness and disease.

Studies have shown parallel developments of increasing environmental toxicity and increasing rates of health challenges in society. This is being reflected in the cancer rate, the rate of Parkinson's, Alzheimer's, diabetes, chronic and autoimmune diseases, as well as neurological disorders.

Identifying the issue is the first step towards change. The major issue in today's health and social crisis is toxicity. All the natural relationships with the environment and surroundings are disrupted and unbalanced. Illnesses develop not overnight but manifest themselves in the body over time. Natural communication and the exchange of information are restricted.

Communication is essential — in the small inner world as in the expanse of the large outer world. A lack of or inadequate communication can potentially destroy long-standing friendships or even cause wars to break out. In nature, we see huge communication networks exchanging information and nutrition. Just look beneath the soil — a network of mycelium extends. Mycelium is much more than just the root of fungi. It connects as a vast communication network between an individual and its environment to exchange information, nutrients, and energy. Human cells communicate as well. Within the small inner world, information, energy, and nutrients are being exchanged. Looking at the outer world's extent, we communicate with our environment. We perceive and absorb emotions, information, and energy. This causes reactions and emotions. Toxic stress disrupts communication, leading to isolation and disharmony. The consequences are health challenges that manifest physically, emotionally, or mentally. But also on a spiritual level — the disconnection to oneself.

The paradigm shift: As the world seemed to flip upside down. Today, I know... It all happened for a reason. Life was meant to be this way — even the uncomfortable moments. And especially the uncomfortable moments, as they make us grow, just like a muscle that needs to be challenged in order to grow. A relaxed muscle does not get stronger.

But all of these building blocks added to a beautiful picture, leading me to an important "New Rule of Wellness": Health issues should instead be related to what is eliminated from our lives rather than what is consumed. Therefore, true health, wellness, and performance don't have to be complex. Achieving optimal health and well-being is within simplicity and understanding. You can find many ideas in my soon-to-be-released E-Book covering sleep, parasites, replenishment, resetting and much more. Connect with me, and I'll pop you in the right direction.

"Cure the Causes" by releasing what is not serving to integrate and bring together the physical, emotional, mental, and spiritual levels in order to allow optimal communication, to free the great potential of the human being, to free the inner wisdom, and to step into true sovereignty. This is a journey. Nothing happens overnight. This is a lifestyle. This is so worth it.

It took me 46 years of life to become the person I am today and discover my new rule of wellness. I stepped out of my familiar shoes and opened myself up to the teachings of the world. Values were put to the test and experienced in a different context. There have been all these experiences,

human encounters, that seem to have nothing in common, but eventually, it comes all together, and you see that all the experiences and people you meet have everything to bring this awareness to the top — having experienced the fall of the wall that had divided Germany for 25 years. A new form of freedom opened up... the world. The world has many facets, different cultures, perspectives, and "secrets".

Uncovering greatness: Over the past four years, at the time of writing this, we have built up a vast network. A network that wants to grow itself. People who want to look out of their small inner world into the great expanse of the infinite universe. Away from science and towards experiencing, feeling, and looking at things holistically. It also marks the beginning of a journey into seeing the human being as something magnificent with superpowers... If you allow it.

For Stephanie Christine, this journey continues.

About the Author

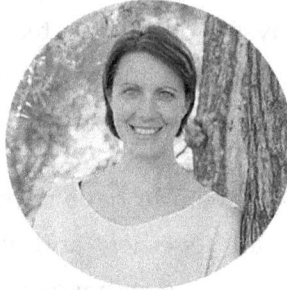

Stephanie Christine's expertise is life; She is a global citizen. Stephanie Christine has a background in nutritional science and Shiatsu therapy. She is a mom, an inspirator, mentor, author and content creator, a free spirit, and the founder of the *Sovereignty Movement*. People have so much potential to unveil. With her work, she provides the space for greatness, by spotlighting the toxicity and the effects of toxicity in today's world, the importance of the body-mind connection and the pineal gland, as well as of sovereignty. Her life-path brought her closer to live in alignment with the natural laws, a holistic way for well-being.

Life has so many question marks? WHY ME?

Her answer: It is meant to be this way. Our life journey is shaped by the lessons learned through our experiences.

Email: stephanie.christine0610@gmail.com
Website: www.stephanie-christine.com
Instagram: @iamstephchristine

Anderson James Daniel

To my childhood friends, I'm Danny, to my Mom, I'm Anderson-James, to my kids, I'm not only Pappa but Jimmy-D, to my gorgeous wife, I'm LoveBug, I call myself the luckiest man alive, and HAVE I got a story to share with the world!

I used to carry the belief, 'words are only words' along with the 'stick and stones' version too, but words can hurt, words are more powerful than actions, and in a cathartic way, *writing the words in this book* and, choosing words in a very specific way to relay my story, is a true sense of wonder to me—I feel it's my chance to do something amazing and to share something amazing too many people would not be able to share.

I have been given a second chance.

I am a veteran, an ex-Naval Aviator, and I had let my role define me, my ego was bigger than any cheque I could write, and the day I died, my whole world changed.

Growing up in a small country town, I had an idyllic childhood where all the farm kids rallied together as best-buds. We fell in love with our child sweethearts and married them as adults. We all had our own homes on our parent's farms and life was wonderful. I became a pilot and was hired by most surrounding farmers as the crop duster, well it turned out I became the ONLY crop duster in our wider area. Then came an idea: I wanted to be more. MORE. This 'life' wasn't enough for me, nor what I could provide my beautiful wife—but this isn't the story I want to tell. My story starts after I died. Prior to that though, I became a generalist pilot in the US Navy to have a different life experience, and yes, we lived on Base, did my time, had three gorgeous children, and then got out, I retired, it was a mutual decision between my wife and myself. We all moved back to the family farm, and life became idyllic for us all.

Unfortunately, my self-importance was brimming over to my own detriment, I became a person I didn't like, my wife called me out on it, as did my childhood friends who most still lived nearby. My self-confidence became a tool for substance abuse.

"He probably has PTSD from the Military," I'd hear townsfolk say (and NO, I didn't).

My self-inflation was a kind of structured confidence; my downfall in hindsight was also my one-sided-conversations, and it was a non-reciprocating lifestyle; it was my lack of perspective, and I thought most rules just didn't apply to me in most areas of my life—I became what is referred to as a tool and, I could see it. My wife loved me, but so much I did and said was apphorable, she called me an A*rse.

Now, I see I WAS that quite a few years later. *Only words*, I used to say back to her, but words can hurt, words are more powerful than actions, I can see upon my continued reflection. Many words, clearly unintentionally, I've blurted out in what I thought was humour that were received as jibes, many words of bad choice were communicated poorly and hurt others beyond my Egos comprehension. I've gone over every conversation in my mind that I can recall having with her, my Sadie, my gorgeous wife I've known from 5th grade, we passed love notes to each other back in 7th grade and sat under the bleachers in 9th grade with pounding hearts and loving each other....and now missing her so much—more than words can ever say. I wish every day I could have the opportunity to re-establish communications with her—the opportunity to revisit conversations and not be such an A*rse!

Maybe one day.

Today, my picture of myself is vastly different. Mother tells me so, and my adult kiddos can see it too—at least we all have each other. I ended up hiding myself behind that inflated Pilots Ego for such a long time. The real me was always there, I made choices I'm not proud of, I did show my real self in my professional career, then learned to hide it away. My *real self* was not to be received or believed. "You can't be that nice all the time," "You are a pushover, you'll never make it here," and "Military Men need to have tougher skin than you have." I threw it back in their faces, changed to what they wanted me to be, and excelled.

The day our world changed

The day started unusually; that should have been a sign, but I thought nothing of it. A bizarre accident was about to happen, and sometimes I feel that surviving against all odds is a defiance of science, withstanding experiences that should have killed me, well, it did actually, but I was revived, and I am alive to tell you.

Our day usually revolved around before sunrise, early farm work, then later a cooked breakfast, and then kids off to middle school on the bus.

None of this happened.

Sadie and I decided to start the morning slowly as we both didn't feel that well, we were all choked up with nasal gunk and hoped the children weren't getting sick, too. We sipped pre-sunrise coffee together and were quite lazy, chatting and laughing. A storm was brewing, and we were intent on listening for any Tornado or Storm developments. The children decided to all stay home, too. Our eldest daughter had a drooping eyelid when she was stressed out, this day, her lid drooped. Our son continued to move at high speed, making pancakes for us all; he felt the healthiest of us all that day. The youngest daughter poured the OJ, intently informing us about the Vitamin C and other Vitamin benefits she had just learned at school. "We need to buy Kiwis, too, they are absolutely PACKED!"

Sadie and I smiled at each other.

Thunder cracked, we rushed to the windows and Sadie and I flew out the front door for a clear view. The wind was coming from all directions, and lightning was striking far off. The hot Sun had heated the ground even that early in the morning, and I could feel the ground- heat rising, with a little humidity in the air.

Sadie and I nodded to each other in unison.

"Get back inside," we both yelled to the children.

I heard a thunderous 'crack', saw the large, majestic, towering native Cottonwood tree receive a lightning bolts direct hit, and the brittle wood exploded—everything went dark—I felt myself falling to the ground. An intense, heavy sensation upon me, I heard the kids screaming, then nothing.

The *nothing* seems to last a lifetime.

Strange things happened next: I felt like I was floating, I *felt* the darkness, and then it changed to a pearly white 'thing', I couldn't see—it was still dark, but a light was somewhere. I could feel myself looking around, but I knew my body wasn't moving. I then felt like I was in a tunnel-like structure and I was traveling through a what looked liked a Galaxy, I could now see Stars dotted everywhere; it didn't feel like I was moving, but just traveling, I 'felt around' for Sadie, yet again I knew my body wasn't moving,

"SADES!!!!" I yelled, then yelled repeatedly, and eventually, she answered me.

"What's going on?" she replied.

"I don't know, can you move, you OK?? I replied, surprisingly not panicking.

"Looks like we are moving, LoveBug, is it a Tornado we are inside of, maybe, where are you, I can't see you, I'm reaching out for you?" she didn't sound panicked either.

"I'm here," she replied now in a whisper, " I can't see you either, I can hear you, I'm reaching out for you take my hand!!"

Suddenly, I didn't know who I was, all thoughts left me, I was floating blissfully, I saw smiling faces, clapping hands, and even what I thought was a welcome sign held by my long-gone Grandmother. I saw multiplicities of me—many of ME's floating around me, like in that Mickael Keaton movie of the same name, Multiplicity—my clones, a kind of coming back to my-many-fragments-of-self. All the 'me's' talking and communicating in a frequently, singing musical notes. I saw purple glowing tree roots, large trees with floating purple branches, what looked like Church bells, a field of Poppies, and random visions—all looked amazing and felt like I was wafting through a movie set. I couldn't hear Sadie, and for a minute, I couldn't even recall who she was, who I was, I didn't know what was happening or what had happened, I didn't know either, I wasn't confused– I just felt light and happy, and a in-love-giddiness feeling overcome me. I felt God. I didn't 'see' anything; there was no booming voice talking to me, and I felt a download of information, an explanation, and execution of His plan—I know, just *knew, to trust, everything would be OK.* Most of us assume we are Finite, but *Infinite* is the truth; to just trust.

The light now was all around me, pearly white mist, a floating around that felt like hours had passed, a bright light, then I felt a sense of gravity, an intense pulling down, moving along inside a thunderous tunnel, then BAM, I felt pain.

PAIN and intense HEAVINIESS.

My vision returned, my hearing returned, and our three kids were in my face yelling at me, the eldest pumping my chest, the other on the phone to authorities.

'What happened?" I looked down as I was pinned under the tree, there was no other damage, it wasn't a Tornado, the house still standing, and the three kids were all OK, I looked to my right, and there was Sadie, lifeless, I realized she was holding my hand while being impaled by a branch. We both had died. I came back, but she didn't. The last thing I heard was, "It's OK, Pappa, stay with us, we've got you." I survived, my wife didn't, and I blacked out.

But don't be sad, my dear readers!

It's now years on, our three kiddos all live with me on the farm, no Tornado ever came and never has, and all the Cottonwood trees have been cut down.

"Anderson-James," my Mother calls to me from the porch— known to us all as Grammy, "It's time," and we are all flocked to the kitchen, treated to Biscuits and Gravy breakfast. The soft bready-biscuits and Grammy's white sausage sauce–heavenly!

We all attend Church together on Sunday, and Sadie's Parents come and stay for the Summer each year. We have created an enormous fire pit ON THE SITE where we both died just off the back porch, and we often sit where I am now ego-less. This is 'my more' to life, I've been gifted a chance to see and experience our children growing up and to become a GranPappa myself. I've become a person I like. Many words surround me, so much love surrounds me now, and I'm so grateful.

I trust. God told me to trust.

My new rule of wellness: When someone shows you their real self, always believe them, and still let them be themselves, for the alternative may not be nice. Is Sadie passing me infinite metaphorical notes? I wonder, for the infinite is possible.

A new existence

It's interesting, isn't it, I do not want to have my story told in a documentary, I don't want to appear on podcasts, and I don't even want to be known as the 'Guy who died and came back,' or 'The After-Death Guy.' I saw an interview many years ago while I was pilot training a 'Near Death Experience Guy,' and I thought, what a load of Cr*p, being a Church-fairing man and all. But I've never forgotten his storyline line of blankness, floating without feeling any movement, various visions, the feeling of elation, light, tunnels, music, then being called back, and a heavy-weight feeling of gravity...you know, I'm sure we all have heard the stories.

It has some merit.

And it's amazing who emerges from the woodwork that resonates with it.

Elaine, whom we went to school with, tells me of the day she drowned and came back. A football fan and friend of mine tells me a story that he has never told anyone about the day he went hunting and shot himself unintentionally, and his experience is similar to mine.

The local community gave me ample support and time to recoup before all the questions started, and I know it's out of pure interest, life, and care, and they all too miss Sadie, of course. The pain of not having her with us will never go away, but it feels like she is with us, it's the reason we never want to leave this house and farm, she so loved it; it was her dream, and she felt an intense connection to the land, and we came back home to live her dream, which we all are doing.

It's quite strange to experience, at the ages we all are now, my school buds come over, a couple has lost their wives too, either age or ill health, we are becoming Pappies and enjoying Grandchildren running around and seeing our kids go through the trials and tolls of rearing a child–the same pains and struggles that we all had. It's a cycle, a journey, an experience, a connection — this thing is called life, and honored to have such a journey. The people you love and meet make it an enriched life. At a younger age, it seems 'life' is all about your career, your business, a wage, money, homes, schedules, and setting yourself up for retirement, it's not about that at all.

Sit with it all.

Take a minute.

TRUST. CONNECT. LOVE. LIVE WITH JOY. EMBRACE
WHAT IS AROUND YOU.

So my second Rule for Wellness is don't let sadness, despair, or
the abuse of substances, or your WORDS, rule you—be
philanthropic, empathetic, and generous as often as you can.

I often watch the Renovation shows where People get advice on
how best to 'fluff their nests' by adding their personalities into
their homes and making a property their forever home—good
on them. I yell at the TV, "Yes, you be you for you!".

Our eldest laughs at me for being 'An-Old-Fella-Now and
Yelling at the TV.'

I see a British family purchasing a French Chateau, and I'm quite
addicted to watching that, too. Seeing them transforming and
growing, creating walled gardens, connecting to their land,
adding their personalities to the many rooms, and experiencing
beauty as a family together—expressing their personalities in
their design, 'Good on you!' I repeat.

I want to be the 'I've found a way to live a healthy life after
immense tragedy Guy.' I'm proud to say my legs were saved in
recovery, and now, to everyone's astonishment, I'm able to be a
'Gym Guy,' I'm fit and have a physique to match any Dad Bod—
no, but to be real, fit and healthy, and making happy and healthy
choices—that's me.

That day, I was shown 'the answers we are all searching for', I felt I was told that the infinite exists, to simply trust and enjoy everything God has offered us without question. To live connected to the land, to live a joyous and fun existence. I now keep chickens and pickle their eggs and give jars of them as gifts, and my great bud owns a bar, he has them as bar snacks for his patrons. I have also planted an American Slicing Hybrid Diamant Cucumber plot they have a perfect texture and the best rinds-to-flesh ratio for pickling. The Grand-kiddos have said they will help me pickle; the older ones will slice, and the younger ones will brine.

I do get asked by many, what now? What to do in 2024?

If I were asked where most people's health focus is at the start of a new year, you'd probably say healthier eating and more exercise. (That's been mine, too, for many years). While that's generally the case and both are important, I think improving gut health is one of the best overall impacts anyone can have on their health and wellbeing, and neurological system too. Hence, my obsession for pickling.

When digestion is good, there's integrity within the gut lining, and a healthy, so many afflictions and symptoms can be overcome — like fatigue, anxiety, headaches, and low immunity. I've enrolled in an online course in Nutrition—never too old to learn new tricks, right? In my now inquisitive opinion, healing and maintaining a healthy gut is essential for optimal health and wellness. Because of its connection with our immune system, hormones, and nervous system function, a healthy gut can profoundly impact how we look, feel, and function and our recovery from injury and depression. Let's face it, most humans go through some, if not all, of these in our lifetime.

You are never too old to live your dreams, either. In recovery, my goal was to get back in the air. I'm now a helicopter pilot for farm usage and fly crop dusting again for neighbors—all those who have supported my family. "Have a great day in your 'office,' Pappa!".

I'm honored to be invited to be involved in this book series, when Dr. Dee reached out, I felt like I still hadn't achieved something, something I couldn't quite put my finger on, and I now feel complete. By being published in a book, I feel I can give them as gifts and also support other amazing humans who need to share something with the world and honor their own Rules of Wellness and life lessons that may be of great value to another person's journey.

You never know who is reading, who is hanging on your every word, whose soul your story has touched, and whose life or perspective you have added a shining light to.

I am Anderson James Daniel; happy, complete, constantly pursuing learning, and a man of my word.

About the Author

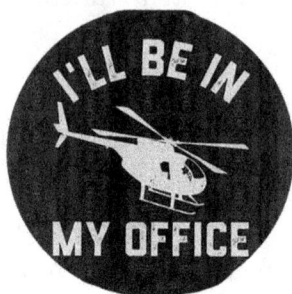

Anderson James Daniel is an ex-military pilot, proud Father of three, and Grandpappy of four. He is an avid fan of health and wellness, is an expert in surviving his life, and expresses that no one is ever too old to learn a new skill.

He died and returned, surviving a devastating lightning strike on the farmland property he calls his forever home. He has stories from the 'other side' and experienced unexplainable things, but now has found his words and voice.

For fun, you will find him flying his helicopter on his family farm, supporting his children and grandchildren, and rising out of his wheelchair into the gym—The hard steel offered a solution for his debility, which saved his mentality.

Email: jimmyd@gmail.com
Instagram: iamandersondaniel

-⌁→

Dr. Quinn Daskins

"Nobody knows anything." ~ William Goldman

You are worthy of all you desire.

We are living in strange times. People are zombified, walking around with their heads stuck in their phones, rechecking their Refrigerator to see if the food fairies have magically delivered something yum straight to their home, iPads have become babysitters, Xbox is a realm of reality and friendships, and other online gaming is creating worlds and alternate universes— it's true to say in my opinion Tech rules. A great example is TikTok; it's dictating current trends and dominates many conversations. I'm increasingly finding that 'nothing is really important anymore,' only the power of our thoughts, connections, and conscious healing… this thing called life is a sort of thought experiment. A matrix of hypotheticals from a logical reason out of a solution to a difficult topic. Where 'things' aren't needed and are only distractions from the truth, the real power lies in our thoughts and intentions, and applying them.

While people plug powerstrips into powerstrips and the mishap is an electrical fire, I've carved a niche out for myself and my partner, where people can power down, live within a space for healing, and time can stand still. I recall from a young age asking my Mother why times have to go so fast, why we always have to rush, and why we can't still do everything but just do it with more peace and with more care for our health; WHY? WHY MOTHER? Why can't we watch the rain fall and splash in the puddles? Why can't we…. With each continued insistence from me, she replied, "Oh, Quinny, ask your father!" Father just nodded, he wasn't emotionally invested in anything while his head was glued to the TV. He did look up at me once that I can recall, "Nothing is important Quinn, I don't know anymore — Live, Die, just exist—-Nothing in-between Quinn until you understand that, go run in the rain."

My partner and I are now Power Down Specialists– how to slow down and enjoy life more.

So, here's how to do it.

The other side: Infinite possibilities with eyes open.

You are worthy of gaining all that you want in life; interchanging energy and shifting focus and perspective and interchangeable with your intentions for the day.

Quantum thought communication - it's instant, not the speed of light as we are currently bound by. Reverse engineering and remote healing, technologies that interface with direct thought, consciousness affecting technology- speed of thought versus the speed of light. Advanced technology and certain technological thresholds go beyond the 'devices' we use. The 3-D reality is lost in this thought experiment, the technology is THOUGHT and biologically interfaced. Technology transfers that can be tapped into–an infinite supercomputer with conscious quantum entanglement and a holographic entity–not just material, but other dimensions with defined frequencies. We live in a conscious quantum hologram. Thoughts are real, so then nobody knows anything really.

This was the day Forensic Medicine was no longer important to me, years ago it was my one hundred percent dream and utmost desire, and within a few hours this day, it meant nothing all of a sudden.

What would you do today if I told you you couldn't fail?

Think about it.

You can start things, learn from them, adjust, set intentions, 'interchange' what you learn so that you succeed, pivot, interface with thought, and change the frequency of the plan if necessary. If I had told my mother that I was going to be a Physician and became one, then quit as I wanted to be of value elsewhere in the world, she would have told me I was mad. I have found a modality and vehicle that I love and can give great support to others.

Forensic Medicine was great, and I loved my colleagues, and if nothing else, met my partner in Forensics, and Voila!

My side: Respect Yourself enough to care.

It was time for me to respect myself more, more than I respected...everything really. I was drowning in my career, I was sick often, and so many other mental things sent me down a rabbit hole of destruction. I 'thought' I was having fun, but I was destroying myself. I had created a world of unhappiness and 'wanted' amazing things to happen, and it was all happening in the opposite direction. But I found many ways to become unrecognizable from this person I'm currently telling you about.

I had to respect myself enough to care.

Are you overthinking it? Not worth it.

Are you still doubting yourself? Not worth it!

Are you always taking the initiative when no one cares? Not worth it.

You will only be seen by the right eyes and the right energy, just enjoy the journey and keep moving, keep planning, and keep creating happiness in your life, amazing things will happen, even after trauma and in times of adversity.

To become unrecognizable by many:

- Wake up early
- Hydrate
- Walk outside daily
- Exercise 5 times a week
- Eat 50g protein per meal
- 8 hours of sleep is a must (one way or the other)
- Cut out all negativity
- EXECUTE THE ABOVE; non-negotiable
- Set up a thought pattern and daily thought practice that will serve you intentions well.

Do less. It's hard to slow down when trying to do a million things.

Be present. It's not enough to just slow down — you need to be mindful of whatever you're doing now. Schedule SLOW TIME. This is a great exercise we do at Retreats. Slow thinking takes time. Slow thinking takes music, frequency, and deep breaths. Slow thinking takes a space of no distractions.

Disconnect.

Focus on people.

Appreciate nature.

Eat slower.

Drive slower.

Find pleasure in anything.

Be boring. Exercise at the same time, eat at the same time, sleep at the same time, get up at the same time.

It's an irony of our modern lives that while technology is continually invented that saves us time, we use that time to do more and more things, and so our lives are more fast-paced and hectic than ever. Life moves at such a fast pace that it passes us by before we can really enjoy it. However, it doesn't have to be this way. Let's rebel against a hectic lifestyle and slow down to enjoy life.If nobody knows anything, then you do you for you, and be you, and do things your way more often than not.

A slower-paced life means enjoying your mornings instead of rushing off to work in a frenzy.

It means taking time to enjoy whatever you're doing, to appreciate the outdoors, to focus on whoever you're talking to or spending time with — instead of always being connected to your iPhone or laptop, instead of always thinking about work tasks and emails.

It means single-tasking rather than switching between many tasks and focusing on none of them.

It means not getting off your desktop, checking the Wifi on your laptop, to then 'having a break' to check your phone Facebook, and Instagram. Can you not see the lunacy in all this? DISTRACTIONS.

Slowing down is a conscious choice and not always an easy one, but it leads to a greater appreciation for life and a greater level of happiness.

Here's how to do it:

1. Do less.

It's hard to slow down when you are trying to do a million things. Instead, make the conscious choice to do less. Focus on what's really important AT THE TIME, and what really needs to be done, and let go of the rest, schedule the rest. Put space between tasks and appointments so you can move through your days at a more leisurely pace. Read more books. Carry a book around with you, get it out at random times and read a few lines.

2. Be present.

It's not enough to just slow down — you need to actually be mindful of whatever you're doing at the moment. That means when you find yourself thinking about something you need to do, or something that's already happened, or something that might happen ... gently bring yourself back to the present moment. Focus on what's going on right now. You can squeeze your muscles (anywhere in your body) to bring yourself back on your actions, your environment, on others around you.

3. Disconnect.

Don't always be connected. If you carry around an iPhone or Tech, shut it off. If you work on a computer most of the day, have times when you disconnect so you can focus on other things. Get up, walk around, schedule in a walk, or swim, or Gym. Being connected all the time means we're subject to interruptions, we're constantly stressed about information coming in, we are at the mercy of the demands of others. It's hard to slow down when you're always checking new messages coming in. Mercy of DISTRACTIONS.

4. Focus on people.

Too often, we spend time with friends and family or meet with colleagues, and we're not really there with them. We talk to them but are distracted—we are there, but our minds are on things we need to do. We listen, but we're really thinking about ourselves and what we want to say. None of us are immune to this, but with conscious effort, you can shut off the outside world and just be present with the person you're with. Connection and community is everything, after all we are advancing our soul experience. Thought connection is vital.

5. Appreciate nature.

Many of us are shut in our homes and offices and cars, and rarely do we get the chance to go outside. And often even when people are outside, they're talking on Tech. Instead, take the time to go outside and really observe nature, take a deep breath of fresh air, and enjoy the serenity. Exercise outdoors when you can, or find other outdoor activities to enjoy such as nature walks, hiking, swimming, etc. Feel the sensations of water and wind and earth against your skin—-do this daily. Jump in the puddles, walk in the rain, sit in the sand, get muddy. Enjoy the sensations.

6. Eat slower.

Instead of cramming food down our throats as quickly as possible — leading to overeating and a lack of enjoyment of our food — be mindful of each bite. Appreciate the flavors and textures. Eating slowly has the double benefit of making you fuller on less food and making the food taste better—-with some great spices and herbs.

7. Drive slower.

Speedy driving is featured heavily in our fast-paced world, but it's also responsible for a lot of traffic accidents, stress, and wasted fuel. Appreciate your surroundings. Make it a peaceful time to contemplate your life and the things you're passing.

8. Find pleasure in anything.

This is related to being present but taking it a step further. Whatever you're doing, be fully present … and also appreciate every aspect of it, and find the enjoyable aspects. For example, when washing dishes, instead of rushing through it as a boring chore to be finished quickly, feel the sensations of the water, the suds, and the dishes. It can really be an enjoyable task if you learn to see it that way. The same applies to other chores — anything actually. Life can be so much more enjoyable if you learn this simple habit.

9. Single-task.

The opposite of multi-tasking. Focus on one thing at a time. When you feel the urge to switch to other tasks, pause, breathe, and pull yourself back.

10. Breathe.

When you are rushed—just pause, and take a deep breath. Take a couple more. Really feel the air coming into your body, and feel the stress going out. By fully focusing on each breath, you bring yourself back to the present and slow down.

Our week starts for us with a 'Blackout' in Peru—-Disconnected from all Tech, most foods whereby we consume a specific culinary diet—-working with amazing trees and herbs, rehydrating, rejigging all our thoughts and actions, detoxing every layer of our being. Anchoring a new energy, it as hard and equally as beneficial and challenging. I'm excited about the next one. Unlocked so many details, deeper into the real me I never thought I would ever be-or even exist. Cosmic download and energy information. NO DISTRACTIONS.

If you can't do blackout, "dopamine fasting" will have a similar physical, emotional, mental, and energetic effect.

The side no one knew.

My now late father's words still haunt me," Live, Die, Exist— nothing in-between Quinn until you understand that, go run in the rain", I think he knew about this thought experiment. He was onto it all along! He knew everything, yet knew nothing at all. What is going to work for you? I bet you don't know until you have a go! And if it doesn't? Not worth worrying about it, move on to the next thing, just keep moving, just keep thinking, and just keep communicating.

Be proud of the work you do, the brilliant person you are, and the difference you make.

"You are the only problem you will ever have, and you are the only solution." ~ Bob Proctor

About the Author

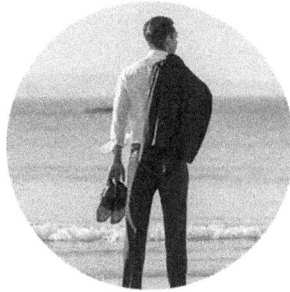

Dr. Quinn Daskins is now a Power-Down Specialist with his partner, reforming their own lives from a hectic pace of Forensic Medicine to the relaxed men they are today.

Back and forth from Canada to Coast Rica, working with some famous names in the manifesting Field; speaking, writing, and teaching; to Power Cleanse and Digital Detox retreats, Revive and Balance Retreats, to OnTrack Retreats and many wellness escapes diving deep into ancient wisdom and natural medical applications.

In their spare time, you will find them in Bali off the beaten track, restoring, maintaining, and protecting natural habitats with the locals, indulging in their own healing practices, and learning new skills.

#highestselfmagnitism

Email: quinndaskins@ymail.com

-WWW→

Deborah DeWet

It started as a love letter to my beautiful twelve-year-old granddaughter. I wanted her to get to know herself better, to fall in love with the beautiful being that she is. I wanted her to know her likes and dislikes, what made her smile, and what she could do if she felt sad. I had a strong desire for her to have a blueprint to help her navigate the adventure of life. She is at the age where we start to become self-aware, developing the ability to state, "This is Me"!

I aim to help her see herself in a positive light and to help train her brain to look for possibilities and instill a love for life.

The love letter I created is a series of questions to help her take time to think and write about who she is. Followed by an uplifting quote and then a prompt so she could write about the best thing in her day. This helps her focus on the good in her day. There is a section for her to write about anything that didn't go so well in her day so she could get that out. Then I asked what she did that made her feel better and what she learned from what happened. By writing the answers to these questions it creates a blueprint, in other words, it starts developing neural pathways that create a new way of looking at life.

We were taught many things in life, but one very big thing we were not taught is how to know ourselves. When most people have taken time to get to know themselves, they have a lot of negative talk going on in their heads. We're rarely taught that life is a journey and a fun adventure. Or that every choice we make leads us down different roads and moves us to explore other paths.

The idea for the love letter that turned into a journal came from a culmination of experiences I had in life. I grew up in South Africa at a time when kids were seen and not heard. That combined with my dad being military, when he told us to do something, we jumped and asked how high afterward. 99% of the time, it was wrong. So we would tie ourselves up in knots, trying to appease or hide.

I married and moved to the United States. I knew there was a better way of parenting than what I had experienced. However, being in a relationship where my nervous system was always on guard did not lead to clear thinking all the time. I used to apologize to my kids for not being the parents they deserved. I knew the parent I wanted to be and felt I was falling short. I couldn't see the whole picture then, but now I realize my kids didn't hold that expectation of me and loved me for who I was. I loved the shift that happened for me. I would get angry with the kids and realize what I was doing, and I would then over-exaggerate the anger and make it comedic. It took the hurt out, and we could laugh together at how silly Mom was being. It was a great healing for me because it stopped the guilt and anger with myself for hurting my children.

There were many times when I could connect with them and express my immense love for them and the magic I saw in them. Perhaps not as consistently as I would have liked. However, to me, they were the most amazingly magical and awe-inspiring people. I wanted them to feel surrounded by love and acceptance.

My oldest daughter, from the age of two always had the same answer to the question I would ask them: "Who loves you the most in the whole universe?' She always replied, " God does, I do, and then you, Mommy."

Fifteen years and three children later I became a single parent. One day, when the kids were away, I remember sitting on the third stair of the staircase, and I started wailing, and I remember screaming at God, "I can't protect them when they are not with me." After a time, the sobbing had subsided, I heard a voice inside say, "It isn't your job to protect them from life. It is for you to be their safe space to return to." "Believe in them so much that it is easier for them to believe in themselves."

I also learned that my job is to model for them what a good life is.

We all learn from experience, and kids watch closely how you are and how you show up in life. Are you showing them how to have a good life? Are you showing them that fun is a wonderful part of life? It doesn't have to cost anything to show them fun. Include them in making a meal together, chase them around the yard, go for walks and talk, find out what interests them, and share your interests with them. Kids want to know they matter to you; they want to make a difference in your life, too. Let them know that when they wash the clothes, make a meal, or take out the trash, they are making a difference in your life; they are your hero. We need to understand and teach them that we are all connected; we rise and fall together, and it begins at home.

So the idea was born that they could continue, whether I was there or not. I set out to build a good life to do just that.

A wonderful tool I was gifted by a friend was to fill the love cup. This entails the child coming to look into your eyes for the love that is there for them. Anytime the child cannot self-regulate, they can come and get their love cup filled. It takes a few seconds, and the child feels seen, loved, and connected. I had taught this to my children, and they had gone to visit their dad.

When they came back, my youngest daughter informed me that she needed her love cup filled, so I asked her which one of the family had helped her. To which she replied that the adults there had no idea about it, and her siblings were not at home at the time. Then she said," Mom, I went to the bathroom and looked in the mirror in my own eyes for the love that is there." What a miraculous moment. I was so proud and so comforted, knowing my daughter did this for herself.

I never remarried when my kids were little. For me, they came before anyone and anything. I also knew I was not in a place to introduce another person into the mix and would not have another complicated relationship to deal with. There was a lot of generational pain in my family, and I was determined to do what I could for it not to be passed down.

I was a volunteer doula - a labor coach. I was always in awe of the new little being lying there in this place that was very new to them. I made a point of welcoming them and thanking them for bringing their beautiful light to the world. There was a thought that I had every time - the marvel of them being tiny, but they're the bosses of their own story. Every decision they make is like a plot twist in their fantastic life movie. This witnessing brought about the knowing that, as parents, we can give them support to allow them to make choices.

I love teaching infant massage in the prenatal classes because I always felt that the parents gain confidence in knowing how to handle their baby and it was a loving and bonding time. I also taught that as parents our job is to help our children become self-reliant. Also, from a young age to let them make simple choices, such as do they want to wear this set of clothing or that set of clothing, thereby building up their ability to make choices and trust themselves.

I worked as a massage therapist, and one of my favorite days of the week was when I went to work with the gymnasts at a friend's gym. Not only did I have the satisfaction of helping alleviate their discomfort, but we got to talking, and it was so exciting to see them light up as they discovered something new about themselves.

Often, I catch myself saying that every child deserves to have parents, like how my kids are parents. I am in awe of how they parent, heck, even I wish they could have been my parents. When my daughter became a parent for the first time, she and her husband told their little one, "We are a team, and we will figure this out together."

I love the shift I see on the planet as more people seek personal growth. As a result, this shift has given rise to a more mindful approach to parenting.

My son was an exceptional father who cherished his children deeply. He adored spending time with his little ones, frequently taking them to the park after a tiring day at work to give their mother some much-needed rest. The children never questioned their father's love, even though he is no longer with us, to this day, they draw pictures and write messages like "My daddy loves me."

My eldest granddaughter, her siblings, and her Mom are my heroes. Although life has thrown my eldest granddaughter some rather large curveballs, she remains kind, generous, and caring. I love seeing her pictures and breathing in the joy of who I know her to be. I want her to see herself through my eyes and know the incredible gift she is to the world.

Often, I lie in bed with my hand over my heart and imagine one of my children or grandchildren in front of me with my other hand over their heart. Then, with my breath, I breathe out my love for them and send it into their Heart Space, and on my inhalation, I receive their love for me. This is one of my favorite nighttime rituals.

With the journal(s) I created, I want a return to the Heart Space, a return to knowing the truth of who they are, and to love everything about themselves. The journal(s) design is to teach them to be gentle when strong emotions take hold and to love themselves even more through it. It will teach them to understand that their emotions serve them as a valuable guide. This will also allow them to understand more clearly what is happening rather than becoming engulfed by the overwhelming force of the emotions coursing through their body.

As most of you who have children know, when you parent your child, you learn to reparent yourself. I am so thankful that there is so much more connection and information. Also, with many families moving away for jobs, there is less pressure to parent the way previous generations used to.

With so much divorce and single parenting, the dynamics have changed. The younger parents are definitely showing a new way of parenting. They need and want a tribe of peers to love and support their family unit, and I love that the grandparents are willing to learn, too.

A beautiful example is when a child doesn't want to give a welcome or goodbye hug to household visitors, the parents and grandparents support it. We don't always know what is going on with these little ones, and if they don't want to hug, it must be for a good reason. This shows them they are supported by the elders in the family. This empowers them to be their own person. This shows them they are valued. What a magnificent trait to develop and take with them on the rest of their life journey.

We live in exciting times where children are seen, respected, and heard, and the parents are fierce advocates for the autonomy and sovereignty of the child.

One time, my son and his family were visiting, and the three little ones were getting rough. I swept up the one who was getting too rough and asked her if she wanted me to take her to the other room. There was so much trust in her eyes when she said yes, and I realized she was looking for a connection. Something in that connection helped her regulate her emotions. In that moment she healed the little girl in me that had felt separated. At that moment, nothing else existed but the love we shared. It was a beautiful bonding experience.

I like the idea that journaling could also become a family bonding experience where everyone could sit together in a room and have a quiet time to journal. People could share if the occasion arose, fostering communication and growth experiences.

I realized how many of us get so caught up in surviving that we forget to look up, we forget that life is about thriving. I wanted to avoid that becoming a habit. That's why I created the love letter to my granddaughter—asking her questions that would lead her to a deeper understanding of herself, finding the great things about her day, and giving her a daily quote to ponder.

One magical outcome of this practice is to train my granddaughter to be on a continuous discovery of "Glimmers." A "Glimmer" is the opposite of a trigger. Glimmers are those micro-moments in your day that make you feel joy, happiness, peace, or gratitude. Once you train your brain to be on the lookout for glimmers, more of these tiny moments will begin to appear.

We all change over a year, and I see the journal as something they could revisit at the beginning of a school year and at the end of that year. This journal is like their growth buddy, helping them become the best version of themselves - like a leveling-up game, but in real life!

Having a blueprint to help navigate the adventure of life is a tool I wish I had when I was young. I'm sure it's a tool you wish you had as well. Understanding how to create joyful life possibilities makes a tremendous difference in the outcome of your "fantastic life movie." I can help you create those life possibilities. You are welcome to connect with me; my email is deborahdewet821@gmail.com.

Also, I have my second edition of "Awaken Your Best Self - Empower Your Inner Self: Nurturing daily practices for self-discovery and mindset shift." One of my favorite elements of this guided journal is the bedtime love letter to yourself. This goes something like this: "Dear Beloved [your name], thank you so much for your kindness to that person today. I appreciate how you live your life from your Heart's guidance. Keep up the great work! Love Me".

I created this second edition so you can journal in real-time in conjunction with your children, creating this lovely atmosphere as a family.

This has great potential to change how families move through life, creating from the Heart. Actions centered on love, appreciation, and understanding of each other. It all starts with the self. By becoming self-aware, we become more aware of others. By learning to love ourselves, we learn to love everyone genuinely. This now becomes a "fantastic life movie" of unity, togetherness and co-operation. The single-household family now turns into a worldwide family where everyone comes together, rises, and evolves.

I love guiding my grandkids to view life through the lens of self-love. One day, I received a heartwarming confirmation from my eight-year-old granddaughter, her sister, she wrote on a Thanksgiving artwork, "I am thankful for myself." These moments truly delight my soul, and instill a love for life.

When creating the cover for the 'This Is Me' journal, my granddaughter requested that the wording be written in cursive. When she saw the final cover, she told her mom she would use it as her profile picture on social media. Upon receiving her "official copy" of the journal, she was excited and couldn't wait to start writing down her thoughts. "This is Me"!

You can find your copy of each guided journal below.

"This is Me: A Guided Journal for Empowerment, Growth & Fun" [Amazon Link - https://amzn.to/3ZNkMXe]

"Awaken Your Best Self - Empower Your Inner Self: Nurturing daily practices for self-discovery and mindset shift." [Amazon Link - https://amzn.to/3T8atvA]

Testimonials

Deborah DeWet has such a peaceful nature within her. I love listening to her just to listen to her heart and the passion that she has within her to help younger kids and tweens, like creating a "This is Me Journal." The kids can use it to become more resilient. Deborah has done this with great intentionality. - Nicolas Goorbarry.

A wonderful journal that focuses a young mind on what matters in life, the one thing that makes a difference in how we live it - how we think and feel. Thank you, Deborah, for creating this sweet journal. It provides positive guidance that we all need! It is a great gift for elementary and middle school kids! Even though I am decades past that age, I concluded that it wouldn't hurt to get one for myself! - J.B.

About the Author

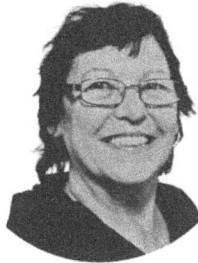

Deborah DeWet is a Mother of three, a Grandmother of Seven, a Wife, and a Mentor. She guides others through the practice of love-centered alignment, journaling, and self-discovery—highlighting the importance and positivity of focusing on our inner being.

She has specialized in Personal Development and Wellness for over 35 years. Starting as a Physical Therapist and Personal Development Training Facilitator in South Africa. She became a Massage Therapist in the United States and simultaneously, she taught for another Personal Development organization while raising three children and prioritizing her personal development journey.

Inspired by her 12-year-old granddaughter, her experience working with gymnasts on their physical and mental well-being, and co-hosting the Happy Neighbourhood Project, Deborah has published guided journals for Youth and Adults.

Residing in Calgary, Alberta, with her husband Lee and two cats, Monty and Ruka, they cherish the city's atmosphere and the nearby mountains.

Email: deborahdewet821@gmail.com
Website: deborahdewet.com
LinkedIn: www.linkedin.com/in/deborah-dewet-55a7841b/

Nicole DuCasse

I grew up in a very traditional Indian family. Education was of the utmost importance, getting straight A's at school was a necessity and the only road to having a successful career and a fruitful life. This message was drilled into me at a very early age, and I now feel was something that laid the foundations for my competitive streak but also ultimately set the seed for my feelings of inadequacy.

Being the older of two siblings, I felt a greater pressure to achieve. My younger sister had a natural flare for dance, and schoolwork came easily to her with little effort. I had to work a lot harder to get similar results. I always felt I was trying to keep up with her, to please my parents, and live up to the dreams they had for me. Primary school was a challenging time. I was culturally different, had different coloured skin, smelly lunches, and an unfortunate lack of sporting skills that made me the last one chosen for the sports teams. I found myself constantly trying to make friends, please the other students, and just fit in.

This challenging trait of pleasing people began at a very early age and continued to manifest in my life as I got older and entered marriage. In Indian culture, the wife takes on the views of her husband. She follows his way of life; her views are consistent with his, and she happily assumes a secondary role to his interests and career. I found myself quickly adopting this place in married life. I feel like I never really got the opportunity to explore my interests, to have a "GO" at life, and to find out who and what I really wanted to be.

There was a fleeting opportunity for this when I completed my Bachelor of Science. Upon graduation, I was lucky enough to secure a highly sought-after pharmaceutical sales role, much to the disdain of my parents, who would have rather seen me settling down in a more secure role in scientific research. This role challenged me; it allowed me autonomy, independence, and healthy competition. I felt like I was beginning to find myself. I was starting to move away from pleasing others and, for the first time, was able to start pleasing myself.

It was only a glimpse. Three years later, I was married, eager, and excited to take the next step. I resigned and dived full steam ahead into my husbands' business, which was a small wildlife education business. I was happy to support him financially and align myself with his dreams and endeavours. That is what I believed a marriage was all about. My parents' disapproval of our business was something that challenged me, and memories resurfaced. I felt like I was disappointing them again. Comparisons with my sister, as she was in a well-paying job in a large organisation, also highlighted this experience. There were times in my marriage when my strength and passion for life came out, however, they were few and far between. Like the time, I decided to participate in a ninety-two-kilometre fundraising walk from the Shrine of Remembrance in Melbourne to the Mt Macedon Memorial Cross. Departing at 10 am from the shrine, we walked through the day and night and ended with a gruelling climb to the top of Mount Macedon in time for the six am ANZAC day service. Of a group of 27 starters, only 6 of us completed the walk. It was a massive achievement and one which I was super proud of myself for completing. However, the pride was short-lived and not a priority in the running of our business. I was oblivious to the fact that I was losing myself again.

I suppose what came next was a pivotal point in the development of myself as an individual. My marriage sadly dissolved, and I found myself alone. My life was in turmoil, and I hated being at home on my own. I had dinner with friends almost every night. I associated myself with people who felt sorry for me and criticised my ex-husband. I was living as a victim, and this behaviour was being encouraged and reinforced by the people I chose to spend time with. We would end the day with copious amounts of red wine, dinner, and trash talk about my ex-husband and how terribly he had treated me.

I found myself in a vicious cycle of self-pity with a victim mentality that was not going to change unless I removed myself from the situation.

One particular night, I left the group knowing that I would not return or see them again.

I had to rebuild my life, and I had to be on my own to do this. Exercise had always been a part of my life, so I decided to start there. I joined a CrossFit gym. I had always believed in surrounding myself with the people I wanted to be, and this is where I found the most positive, supportive, and encouraging community. I started viewing competition in a healthier way rather than as a comparison between my sister and I. I learned to compete with myself and be 1 % better than I was the day before.

This Facebook reel, which has had over 1.5 million views, sums it up perfectly. It is a movement that professional cross-fitters can perform quite easily.

https://www.facebook.com/reel/3097126947265757?fs=e&s=TIe Q9V&mibextid=0NULKw,

However, I was determined to do it as well, and I did just that. I was achieving for myself, not as the partner of someone who was successful. I was making my two girls proud as well as instilling in them a love for health and fitness.

Concurrently, I joined a health and wellness network marketing company. Personal development is prioritised, as well as relationship-building skills. I was being challenged again. I was educating people on the benefits of pure therapeutic ketones as an alternative fuel source, and I was motivating people to change their lives through movement, diet, and mindset. I was good at what I did and moved up in the company quickly. My way of thinking was first challenged in my role here. They encouraged us to do our own research and to look outside the mainstream media for alternative health answers.

I felt very conflicted by this at first. I had been brought up in a home where the news was the most important part of the day, and we would all sit and watch it in silence. It was gospel. Doctors were viewed as Gods. Whatever they said, we did without question. I had also finished a four-year science degree, and some of the research I was uncovering with Pruvit was contradictory to what I had studied. The deeper I dug, the more I realised the connection between Big Pharma and dollars. They needed people to be sick in order to keep making money. Healthy people were of no value to them. If people could heal themselves with diet and exercise, these companies would become redundant. The research that was taught to us at university was not necessarily the truth. It all depended on which company paid the most money, as this was the paper that would get published and then taught to us. I felt robbed, hollow, but also angry. It was so unfair; people were being given misleading information by authoritarian figures who were supposed to be helping them. Instead of becoming healthier, the population was becoming sicker. From this point, I vowed to educate myself on all alternative therapies and medicines. I had done a full 360 degrees, and I was passionate about my decision to help others with a holistic approach to life.

I love learning, and reading has always been a passion of mine, one that sadly dropped off while I was married due to lack of time. I was eager to get back into this, and one of the first books I read was 'Rich Dad, Poor Dad' by Robert Kiyosaki. This book had a profound impact on my life. It reinforced the fact that I could create a life for myself and my girls with my online business. I felt confident that I should pursue my dreams despite the lack of excitement from my parents about my new employment choice.

One of my favorite quotes, which I live by, was told to me at a self-development workshop I attended very early on in my business: Marry the Process, Divorce the Outcome. This is extremely powerful and something I wish I had lived by in my earlier years. My life was always about working towards something, getting the ultimate job, having the perfect family. Now, I live my life in the totally opposite way. I'm in love with the process and do not care about the end result. I am grateful and enjoy every single day. I no longer grind through the week, only living for the weekend. I look forward to every day, and I am truly grateful for the life I have created.

At the start of this year, I decided to give weightlifting a go. I felt like I needed a break from CrossFit and a new challenge. It was tough, but I enjoyed using my brain again. There was also an irrational fear associated with it, which had prevented me from taking it up earlier. The mere thought of walking out onto a lifting platform in complete silence, except for my weightlifting shoes hitting the polished wood, made my stomach clench and my breath catch as if I was going to pass out. This was comparatively insignificant after everything I had faced in my life so far.

Therefore, it was something that I had to do.

Divorcing the outcome and marrying the process was at the forefront of my mind during training, and I enjoyed every moment. I set myself up for success and did everything I could to be ready for competition day. This included monitoring and maximising sleep consistency and duration, maintaining adequate daily hydration, targeted clinical Pilates for Glute activation and strength, a tailored nutrition program with

: The New Rules of Wellness

macro tracking to ensure the weight loss was body fat and not muscle mass, and specific vitamin supplementation to support my training goals. I felt great leading up to my competition, but as it got closer, I had to face my fear, and that needed some mental help. I listened to "Clean up Your Mental Mess" by Caroline Leaf and realised what my real fear was. I was scared of letting my coach down after all the effort he had put in. Dr. Leaf said that many of our fears could stem from childhood experiences, and my people-pleasing traits were resurfacing. I acknowledged this and where they were coming from but decided to reframe my thoughts. I had already done the work, and my coach was already super proud of me. What I was feeling about the comp was not anxiety and nerves but, instead, excitement to show everyone what I could do. This simple shift in mindset was all I needed. I was successful and ended up with two equal personal best lifts on the platform.

I was also the oldest female to qualify for the weightlifting finals later in the year. More importantly, I enjoyed the experience and was able to overcome a deep-rooted fear of mine.

I feel like I am in a great place right now. I am financially stable, I get to inspire, motivate, and help people, and I have plenty of time to train, travel, and have other interesting experiences. Sadly, there is something missing in my life, and that is my beautiful younger daughter, whom I think about every single day. The last time I saw her was when she was 11 years old. She is now 17 and has had no contact with my family or myself since then. It is heartbreaking to think of all the time we have lost, the milestones in each other's lives missed, and the memories we have been unable to make. I get comfort from knowing that she is well looked after. Aside from that, there is nothing more that I can do except hope that one day, she will feel ready to allow us back into her life. For now, I need to put the sadness in a drawer and close it. I need to live my life and enjoy it with my older daughter. She is a real go-getter, brilliant, strong and intelligent.

She inspires me daily to take life by the horns, never give up, and never stop believing in myself.

You can do anything, MUM!!!

I am very grateful for the impactful changes I can make in people's lives on a daily basis with my social media content. I love to share my experiences with my audience in a raw and honest way on these platforms. My business kickstarted it all. I learned how to share information and education to a broad audience utilising the Facebook and Instagram platforms as well as my scientific training.

In this Facebook live

https://www.facebook.com/nicole.ducasse.79/videos/10772397 99138645/?mibextid=cr9u03

You can see the benefits of utilising ketones as a fuel source as opposed to carbohydrates. I was able to connect with like-minded individuals all over the world. This was an incredibly empowering experience. My business now ticks away organically and provides me with a residual income. It is enlightening and encouraging people to look outside traditional medicine for health options. I love to keep up to date with anything new in the health and wellness space and am a willing guinea pig to try them out. I'm currently waiting on the delivery of a grounding sheet, looking forward to my first session of sound healing, and excited to be working with an NLP coach for mindset in competition. I am not only obsessed with experimenting with myself but also with tracking the results so that I can share them. I wear a Garmin watch on my left wrist and a whoop band on my right wrist. Tracking sleep and recovery is super important to me for my training, but also so that I can enjoy the best quality of life. I also use social media as a daily reminder to share the simple tips I live by. Drink a minimum of 3 litres of water. Ensure you go to bed and wake up at the same time each day (at least within an hour). This is more important than the duration of your sleep each night. To move your body every day and to live in the moment every single day. Life is just too short not to.

I have created a life by design that allows me to work 3 hours a day as a carer.

This is a super rewarding experience and one in which I have been able to utilise my own business skills to help my client start up her own gourmet hamper business. The rest of the day is free for me to train for my next weightlifting goal and to explore other interests. I want to try everything in life at least once. I have a dream to join the Victorian Masters Weightlifting team. I have purposely not given myself a deadline for this as I want to truly enjoy the process and divorce the outcome.

My flexible working arrangement also allows for my penchant for travel. Travel has been pivotal in the development of my independence. I would never have imagined I would travel alone. When my marriage dissolved, I thought that was also the end of travel for me. But it was a passion of mine and, therefore, another fear I had to face.

I found a company for solo travellers specialising in the forty to fifty-year age group, and I have never looked back. I am so grateful to have visited 15 countries in the first 12 weeks of this year. It started with an amazing trip to Scandinavia to see the Northern Lights. I visited Norway, Finland, Denmark, Sweden and Iceland. The next trip was to Jordan, and the last was to Vietnam and Cambodia. This April, I have an adventure planned to the Galápagos Islands, the Amazon Jungle, and Macchu Picchu. Look at me go! I am so proud of who I have become and my attitude to life.

Time is the most valuable commodity and something that is always at the forefront of my mind as I wait and hope for the day when I can reconnect with my youngest daughter. Love you always and forever. Once time is gone, you cannot get it back. To enjoy the most quality time on this earth, health is paramount. I want to inspire people to be healthy and to be the best possible versions of themselves so that they can have more quality time on this planet. I want to remind people of the importance of time and help them to live every moment of their lives to the fullest.

Living for today, as tomorrow is not guaranteed.

About the Author

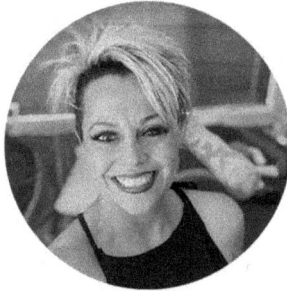

Nicole DuCasse is a self-proclaimed biohacker. She has graduated from the University of Melbourne with an honours degree in Microbiology. She also has a certificate 3 and 4 in fitness, nutrition and personal training. A Spinning certification as well as a crossfit level one accreditation. Her passion for self-improvement and drive to help others, led to the establishment of her own online health and wellness business, which has been successfully changing lives for the past 8 years.

She is an avid CrossFitter and masters weightlifter, with a dream to eventually qualify for the Victorian Masters weightlifting team. She lives in Victoria with her little man Archie (a very spoilt 7-year-old Chihuahua) and has two amazing daughters, 19 and 17 years old, who inspire her daily. The mantra she lives by is "Marry the Process, Divorce the Outcome".

Email: crosskore@gmail.com
Facebook: Nicole Ducasse
Instagram: @coachnicduc

-WW→

Mountain Man Lawrence DZ

My New Rule of Wellness: Ask for what you want, for it's already there in Nature.

Hi, I'm DZ, and Yes, I'm a Mountain Man. I live way out in the wilderness, alone, in a set of Mountain Ranges in the Northern Hemisphere, and I don't want to be found.

I have no electricity or modern things, I'm not keen on people most of the time, I'm happy and peaceful where animals and lakes are my neighbors, and I live off the land and fend for myself. Yes, I have dreadlocks, yet sometimes I shave my head. I bathe in the lake, swim in the lake, eat from the lake, and in winter, ice fish on the lake. You may ask me how I am writing this; I'm writing this because Dr. Dee reached out to me and wanted me to share my experiences with the world. I go into a town every once in a while, and one of her friends on Facebook is someone I buy supplies from, she mentioned me, the timing was immaculate, an introduction was made (Zoom interview),

155

and I stayed in the town a few days so Dr. Dee could extract a story from me to share. Here it is.

My life motto, 'Ask for what you want, for it is already there in Nature,' aligned directly, she asked. I was there and said yes, and I am so honored and pleased my 'normal life' will be shared with the globe, as I realize my *normal life* will be an adventure, or torture, for others, for people to read and experience too. Dr. Dee said she was a fan of the 'Alone' TV series (clearly, which I've never seen). Still, as she explains the harrowing occurrences on the show, the contestant's experience, I resonate with what she said about general life living in those altitudes and wilderness.

Happy to share.

Dee: How did you become this Mountain Man DZ, were you a Mountain kid?

DZ: I grew up with my Father hunting, my Mother died, and my father raised me. He is a skilled trapper. Nothing tragic ever happens, really, just life. "That's just life, Son," Pappa told me. He taught me everything I know today, when he died, I decided to go to the hills. I never came back. I'm not a squatter, I own some land in my own right and choose to live there, way away from everyone else. I cut my own materials, built a dugout shelter, and created a bed, oven, and running-water system— its a comfortable home for me, and it's all Winter secure also. I forage, hunt, and grow all my food, built a good meat-smoker, and a larder for Winter food storage, which is very effective. I'm busy all the time, there is always something to do, and it's not just survival, but my home and my life. I love my life. I have great fun and create my happiness. The rain is my music. The lake in early August has big toothy predators lying beneath- Lake Trout, or Bull Trout is a good meal.

Dee: Do you keep any books where you live, DZ?

DZ: Absolutely, I love reading. I'm looking forward to you posting this one so I can read everyone's stories too, honored to be among other amazing people. Some of my books have been destroyed by rain; I keep my special ones in leather cases. I keep them in a space that is a moderate environment near the oven and store them upright like any other person does I assume. I like Westerns, medical books, and poetry like Edgar Allen Poe. I have one of his literary critics' gothic books, 'Castle of Otanto' — very rare.

Dee: Tell us about your incident fighting the elements, how does nature provide even in extremes?

DZ: My elevation is high. Somedays are misty; some days shape up to be nice days…these days, I bathe, and when I hit that cold water, I scream like a child. The cold water gnaws at you, you lose your manhood in seconds, and the wind picks up, telling me to get out. I have a solid home, a perfect cabin dug into the side of the hill, protection from the elements in all seasons. This is living in the wilderness and interacting with nature, which few people experience. I get things done while my energy is high and then rest up. Nights are tricky, and sometimes a good sleep is not: Warm and dry, Water and food are the key. Protein is also vital to consume daily. Sometimes, my fishing lines become rat nests; I'm a skilled trapper and hunter.

Chef DZ's cooking cuisine is Bull Trout Head Soup: Water, head, chopped Solomon Seal Root and Slimy Spike Cap (Mushroom), simmer, and the fish head skin is great. Smoking meat takes 24-48 hours but attracts the Bears. Storing my smoked meat is vital, keeps away the animals (as they can't smell it fresh or cooking) and lasts longer in my larder. I built a boat, perfected it so it's not tippy, and you need kickback so it holds you up—I have a furr frame and a tarp, and made Oars. Dependable and safe so I'm not limited to bank fishing. Winter is months of snow cover, your everyday white stuff, and this is when life gets different. Wet snow is the worst, packed snow is easier to deal with, and then snow storms and snow drifts don't tend to affect me whole bunch due to my choice of location other than a snow bank forms. Bears tend to wander but don't come into my camp, have never shredded anything of mine all the years I've been living here. I have many traps set around the perimeters of my camp, and I have a Drahthaar hunting dog that doubles as a ski-jor in Winter, and triples as my best buddy too—Boone. Nature provides plenty of water, if not I melt the snow.

The Mushroom Incident

I'm now a skilled farmer, but sometimes by trial and error. There are over 500 mushrooms native to the Northern Territories. They love growing under the Conifers, Balsams, Jack Pines, Alders, and Tamarack, and most edible ones have a sister-like non-edible or psychedelic counterpart. Certain mushrooms grow continuously throughout the season, we call them 'flushes', and I'm cultivating an area that I re-visit after harvesting. I am farming Morels. 'True-Morels' and 'False-Morels' look similar, one is the edible variety, and one is poisonous. Yes, I know you can tell what's coming: nausea, vomiting, abdominal pain, diarrhea, headache, cramps, and I couldn't function. Boone was worried about me–luckily didn't last long, and confusion didn't arrive. I dare say there were moments I was questioning and confused over what I had done to myself. Boone wasn't sick, what did I eat that he didn't? False-Morels look like lumpy brown, grey, white, or red caps with a brain-like wrinkled appearance and pitted surface going INWARDS. True-Morels also look brown, grey, white, or red caps, bulges coming OUTWARDS. See my initial dilemma? They look nearly identical to an untrained eye. The True-Morels stand up like a pine cone and are symmetrical, False is more like a non-symmetrical brain. My eyes are now trained, and my farming skills are impeccable.

The Mountain of Uncertainty

Living on a Mountain is uncertain, yet it seems that most people's life is also uncertain. So our lives aren't all that different in reality. Some of us have developed habits and mental models to reduce or eliminate kinds of stress, for the majority of people, I'm sure it is the level of management of this stress that is taken into account; uncertainty can be off the charts and out of your hands, or it can be skillfully negotiated and negated....and uncertainty is a primary cause of stress. I sometimes face a dark and murky wilderness, and other times, a light and sunny heavenly landscape and nightscape. The full moons are particularly gorgeous I look up at it from my rugged front porch. Planning is everything. Imagine the stress I would have—and possibly perish—if I didn't plan for Winter? There are many mental models, exercises, and tricks to help reduce uncertainty.

You draw a map, a 2 x 2 grid; **what is important** and **not important** on one axis, then, **I know**, and **I don't know** on the other axis. Place all the things on our minds in certain relevant boxes. For example, Important: Harvesting, protein collection, water pump repair, New roofline, new ski. Then concentrate on the boxes; **what is important** and **I Know.** Your map will become clear, and you can plan the next steps until the season changes.

My life runs by seasons and full moons.

The **I don't know** and **not important** boxes you can increase your learning and new skill development or put those things off that aren't important until they become either important or fun to do but not entirely necessary for life processes. Navigating life processes doesn't have to be difficult, even when living in extreme environments. The mind is an extreme environment. People believe I don't get lonely, I like my own company, I have Boone, and I like living in my own mind.

The Lost Hiker

I woke up to the voice of a young man—shouting. He could see the smoke from my fire and headed my way. Now, it's a no-go-zone around my camp due to specifically placed concealed animal traps, and my area is a good day's hike in a certain direction to civilization. He was lost and about to fall victim to one of those traps. He was in poor condition, and since he 'visited me,' we have met in town a couple of times over the last couple of years to catch up. A Bear had slashed him, his toenails blackened, and had become lost on his 'backcountry splashes' hike.

"Lakes, Mountains, Vistas," he said was the attraction once he spent a few days with me recovering. His hiking and camping friends headed back, and he was to stay just one more night and head off in the direction they went at the first break of daylight. He headed the opposite way without noticing.

It was strange to have someone else in my camp. He was grateful to be alive and couldn't believe his luck in finding me, couldn't believe I lived here by choice, "In this hell-hole," a stark change from his attitude of the delightful tune of his 'backcountry splashes adventure' of four days ago.

"That's just life, Man," reiterating my father's sentiment.

"I couldn't live without Fries" was one of the first things he said once delirium had passed. He spoke of walking forever with the world starting to fall off either side of the now arrow escarpment—tough hiking—famous area for bio-diversity and being a student was very mind-averted and lack of concentration, oblivious to the advancing wildlife, advancing sunset, and advancing dense area than he had recalled on his way in—Very dangerous recipe. The next day, he said he couldn't believe how windy the earth could get.

He admires me; no company, no wife, no kids, no 'home' as he knows it, no "people" anywhere—tough enough to handle the wild.

"Nothing like a god bushwacking!" I got him laughing, and he survived, so my 'Medicine-Man' skills are adequate, too.

"What do I call you?" He said the day I was taking him into town; he was well enough to put those hiking boots back on.

"DZ, that will do, you are now my friend."

"I owe you my life, DZ," he replied. " I will never forget your kindness."

"Owen," his name was, "You need to learn to start living with nature, not fighting it for survival." Everyone I've ever met seems to be in survival mode, not thrive mode.

"Ask for what you want, for it's already there in Nature, I won't forget it, I promise," said Owen, and he hasn't either. I met him these past few days while I've been 'consulting' while Dr. Dee writes about me. He bought me some of his favorite French Fries. "Might be better than that Liver Soup water you made me drink!!!"

Fresh signs

I see fresh signs, "Let's see if we can catch something, Boone."

It's late in the morning, and they are probably bedding down. Deer. There is a Buck right there, staring right at me. I stare back, Boone doesn't move a muscle. *Don't spook, don't spook.* It's gone behind a tree. Cross my fingers; the larder needs to be filled. I feel myself take each breath, sounds so loud when you are trying to be quiet. "Ohhh, Lord, Thank You for your gifts". I shout out as Boone runs over. Hunting is something I've done my whole life, being self-supported by what the land provides is truly a blessing. There are major predators here, and the last thing I need is a Bear coming in to steal it. I get the job done, keep it from spoiling, and organize dinner tonight—always eat the heart first–it's significant to me—Boone licks his lips.

Drum and Leather Tanning

There are times when one wants to sing and dance. So, early on in my solo-living I tanned my leather from my catch, stretched it, tooled it, and made my own drums. Hairblades and certain tools are essential and I made mistakes, and now I've perfected my art. It's the attitude of applying myself to succeed in what you do. I have a great few drums, and Owen and I enjoyed the time singing around the fire, he said that moment changed his outlook on life, too. You do not have to be perfect or even great, just give it a go if that is what you want to do. Boone and I sing and dance at night in the darkness, it's great. I drum in the back where my bed is, and softly as a mediation, sometimes Boone kicks me in his meditative sleep—true relaxation, vibration, and frequency.

Dee: Thank You, DZ, it's been totally amazing chatting and sharing with you, any last words you want to share with the world?

DZ: Healing. You have it in you to heal whatever needs to be healed, and all the tools are in Nature. Either get out it more or utilize it well, for it is supposed to be lived in and looked after in return. Those few days with Owen really changed my perspective on how civilized people live in such a false world.

(to me). Illusions of greatness and success, the falseness of 'surviving,' and toxic relationships with obsessions—ditch it all.

Dee: And Leading from the heart, DZ?

DZ: Always—leading from the heart—the only tool anyone needs. When you lead from the heart, every solution is found. Land connection—nature takes over, so learn to live harmoniously with her, and she will provide. Just connect.

In the grand symphony of life, fun, rain, nature, and happiness are the most beautiful melodies.

Author Bio

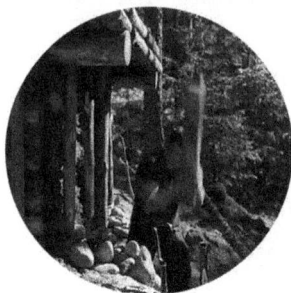

Mountain Man Lawrence DZ, known as DZ to many, lives in the wilderness of the Northern Hemisphere Northwest Territories, way out up——somewhat near—The Great Slave Lake, Canada, where Nature provides all for him.

In the grand symphony of life: fun, rain, nature, and happiness are the most beautiful melodies.

He lives— he lives well, with the need for nothing more than he already has.

He says thank you for reading his story, and he hopes you can find gratitude for all you have too without the poison of 'want'.

-⋁⋁⋏→

Marie Agnes Elson

"If there is a panacea, or cure-all to life, it is self-love."
~ Paul Solomon

This day starts like no other day; we are moving house. As you read this, the move is taking place—long-held dreams are coming true. I had always wanted to live in a 'Two-Story-White-House-By-The-Sea' (this line I would reply within many conversations over the years when I was asked), Keith, my husband, and I, via the love and dedication of our daughter, Nereda, are moving at long last to a dreamy Rosebud Villa at the age of 89!!

However, this is not the story I will tell you today; it begins with a left-of-centre career change that emerged out of nowhere over 28 years ago.

First, Authorship

I had collected many things over the years, from my global travels and varied professions in my younger years to my parenting years when we took our Daughter on many holiday adventures, to my years of house-sitting assignments: Medical books, Self-help books and publications, Psychology and Health, Natural Medicine and Homoeopathic books, many thought-provoking practices of Cherishing, Meditation, Yoga and so much more.

Great inspiration I have gained via thousands of interesting publications; I have loved Dr. Wayne Dyer's works and teachings (Author and Motivational Speaker), Ram Dass (Spiritual Leader and Guru), Louise Hay (Metaphysical Lecturer) and all the brilliant work of Hay House, Paul Soloman (Meta-Human Ideals, Healer, Prophet, Minister, Humanitarian), Suzi Holbeche (Spiritualist and Crystal Healing Specialist), The Findhorn Foundation and Steiner Schools (New Age Living and learning), Dalai Lama (Advocate for Peace and Freedom - Buddhist), and many community spiritual groups, communities, and publications—so many things have influenced my magical life.

I have also been in a place of influence myself assisting many people along their journey of life, discovering their full potential, creative powers of self growth, life enrichment and pure divine guidance.

I have produced my own works and publications, 'Marie's Work and Play', 'Stardust And Grace Co-Authored with Dr. Dee, 'I Choose To BE Happy- Happiness Comes From Within'' to be released by The House of Wellness Publishing in 2024, and 'My Mind is Ever New'--a series of Puzzle books with metaphysical quotes, ' —look out for them, or contact Dr. Dee to orgaise your copies.

So, where did I start when Dr. Dee asked me if I could offer some 'New Rules of Wellness' inspiration to those who need it? I start with my all time number one— Positivity.

We can all feel, at times, there is an invisible blockage. Something is stopping you from experiencing 'life,' your happiness, peace, abundance, joy, love, success, and health— whatever it is, it's there and can be a life changer if you address it. Dis-ease can be reversed simply by reversing mental patterns knowing that the point of power is only ever in the present moment; from there you can create your own magic. Imagine if I told you that its possible to take life in perfect balance?

Complaining: does it get you anywhere?

Overthinking: does it get you anywhere?

Stuck in monotony; does it get you anywhere?

Negative thinking: does it get you anywhere?

Repeating what doesn't serve you well: does it get you anywhere?

Obsessions: does it get you anywhere?

Coveting: does it get you anywhere?

Procrastination: does it get you anywhere?

Ignoring, and Denial: does it get you anywhere?

Stressing; does it get you anywhere

These things DO get you somewhere, to the location no one ever really wants to go—but you can end up there anyway—ill health. It's time to venture inward towards your own awakening. Accept that you have full power and accept that loving and approving of yourself herein lies the magic for a united and balanced life.

My New Rule Of Wellness: To be positive, to breathe, to be happy, to be loved, to feel safe, to be peaceful and to feel a sense of accomplishment. Choose to experience the sweetness of today—the sweetness of right now.

Find a supportive practice that offers you Peace, Happiness, Abundance, Joy, Love, Success, Health, and, most of all, something that has you *feeling* that you are accomplishing things.

A supportive practice will vary from person to person, for some, it is the Gym that has saved their lives, some are getting out of the relationship and starting a new way of living with new activities, for some, it is a change of routine, or travelling, or ticking off a bucket list item.

Start with your breath. It's always available; it's essential to life, it's free, accessible, and dependable—the perfect place to start.

Find something to get excited about— in the now.

Find something to make you laugh—in the now.

Find people to communicate and commune with–in the now.

Find a way to 'notice' and pay attention to what is going on around you—NOW.

Feel the breeze outside, see the birds and insects, listen to the rain, sip the water, and feel its hydration. Be interested in your health—self-care and self-love. Find natural ways, and read each day—It's always a good time to pick up a book. (Why don't you keep one in your purse?) Educate yourself on something new. It's never too late to learn something new, never too late to start something new either. Or move house—look at us today!!

When was the last time you picked a flower and smelled it?

See yourself taking the action steps; your new self will thank you for it.

Repeat: "I choose to fill my world with joy. I love and approve of myself".

I close my eyes, and instead of darkness, I see sparkles, lights, and colours—it's quite magical. I sit and do my 'Universal-Love-Breath' tune-up technique; this has always given me a pick-me-up during the course of my life whenever I needed it—especially invigorating if you feel rundown, fatigued or 'a little-off'.

It's about setting an intention for what you desire to realign.

Visualise a large GREEN energy plasma ball–it's crystalline with shiny, shimmering suspended particles. Imagine inhaling the green glistening liquid and telling your system to detoxify anything that doesn't serve you well. Feel that your 4-body-system (Spiritual body, Mental Body, Emotional body, and physical body) in the restoration process, and trust whatever balance you need will be restored.

Today is a new day; you deserve to be more than how you have been treating yourself lately. What can you do today to create more happiness, joy and accomplishment —today? We cannot become what we need by remaining where we are. When you change, everything changes around you. Enter yourself into a new age of energy, and your experience will deepen—answers come when you let go.

If this message finds you, this is meant for you.

Moving into the next version of yourself takes new capabilities and new experiences, boundaries will be tested, but you will be more spectacular when limitless possibilities are there. Push through and change a little. The past is now behind you, only NOW exists—and embrace new possibilities. A newness is now available to you, follow your faith.

This is your time to shine and see the sparkles too.

Secondly, left-of-center career change that emerged out of nowhere

It was never my intention to become a housesitter, I "fell into it"!" My old boss of many years, after their retirement, purchased a small farm and therefore suggested I come to mind the farm while they go on vacation to their holiday Villa in the tropics, and in turn, I too could have a holiday for a heated northern exposure vacation too if I liked. "Yes, please!"

It all snowballed from there really—within a year, I found myself booked out for 18 months in advance for other friends, and referrals, and years on, I was booked 4 years in advance. I then began to take special requests, and what a joy it's been. Some of these stories I share below:

Bed and Breakfast Joy

Bed and Breakfast: Mount Dandenong Ranges, Victoria, Australia.

I did have a choice when first approached for the job: Mind the house, dog, garden, 6 chickens and be paid a weekly fee, or run the guesthouse as my own business in return for the takings. I chose the latter and went back for many years to come, and absolutely loved every minute of it—so many wonderful guests and experiences, and My grandchildren would visit, and we went for a ride on the local scenic Steam Train, "Puffing Billy" just down the read from the guesthouse—great memories as we took our own daughter on Puffing Billy 40-odd-years prior when she was 3 years old.

One Saturday evening there was a phone call for accommodation, luckily I had a cancellation. The family had gone for a drive in the hills, loved it so much, and wanted to stay. They arrived with takeaway food and insisted I join them for the meal around the open fire. I had been their 'last resort' call—thankfully it all worked out. The guesthouse usually serves Devonshire Tea (fluffy Scones, Jam, and Whipped Cream), homebaked cakes and a friendly "hello" from Jenna the Blach Labradore, so I would match that sentiment 'on my shifts' at the B&B.

Beau Boy

Before taking a new client, I'd organise an appointment to meet them, and their pets and assess the surroundings to ensure compatibility. 'Beau Boy' watched me ascend the drive. He was sitting Sergeant-Major style on guard, after studying me, then greeting me with the biggest tail wag—his rear-end nearly wagged off. That was it—love at first sight.

"Aren't you gorgeous," I replied to his endless rump-wagging. His owners arrived home and he placed his body in front of me, sideways, "My goodness, he is guarding you from us now!" My note to 'tuck Beau in at night and cover his legs as they stick out and get cold', I adhered to lovingly without question attending to Beaus each need, and in return, Beau Boy and I are forever friends.

Roast Dinner

It was 1999, my granddaughter then was 3 years old. She announced she was getting a ".....Mation Dog—and her name is Spice". With such excitement and enthusiasm, Spice enters all our lives, and they all end up moving to Queensland to Tropical beachfront living—an absolute Paradise. I then travel up to Mackay not only to visit but to mind Spice too, at Sunset Bay. Spice, too, was in paradise, she would visit the neighbours and be given treats. I think she overstepped the mark one day when she came home with a complete roast (obviously, take out to thaw on the bench) I am sure was not a gift. Maybe the one family in the street having an unexpected vegetarian dinner that night.

The Queens Knitting

I minded a lovely Staffy named Queenie, no wonder her name was Queenie she lived in the most palatial dog house you could imagine. Her life companion was a British Blue cat named Hamish, and these two lived a playful life running all over the house and chasing each other. One evening after dinner they were racing happily, then Hamish came and joined me in the kitchen. Queenie continued her racing, then an unusual quiet enveloped the room. S-I-L-E-N-C-E. I entered the loungeroom — SHOCK HORROR! My knitting that had been on the coffee table was now totally undone — each stitch of wool was wound around furniture, miles of wool around most pieces of furniture — the Queen had done her un-knitting very well.

Pot-Plant-Pussy-Cat

Lulu became a garden cat — she loved to sleep in flower pots and her favorite place was the wheelbarrow. The first time I minded the house she gave me much angst. The gentle, loving pussy cat was really an imposter; she had attitude and a bossy temperament, she lived over the back fence, but, as she insisted that she wanted to live on 'this side' of the fence, the two neighbours agreed on this arrangement (Cats tend to do things their way). The house was full of antiques, valuable ornaments, crystals and other treasures. Lulu would jump on the cabinets covered with delicate things, I held my breath imagining the ensuing CRASH and SMASH, but no—she was nimble-footed and wound herself around contorting here body before she jumped down—what a 10/10 performance! A Double-trouble-imposter actress—really a beautiful, gentle soul.

Friendly Farm

A distant relative of mine asked if I would mind her friend's farm, I agreed to investigate the possibility— 2 dogs, 2 horses, 5 cows, several chooks and an Owl up a tree—the Owl up the tree sealed the deal for me.

Tilley and Tommy, the dogs, were a total delight, we walked in the fields and they fended off all the pestulant European rabbits. All the above listed was there too, including a field full of Kangaroos at Sunset and Sunrise and a winding creek passing by the backdoor. Such a "fun" farm it was—I fed the horses fresh carrots and the cows came running at the sight of me—bellowing at me, wanting their fare share of treats, too. When I fed the chicken as they were free-ranging on the back lawn, they shared their meal with the Doves, Wrens, Cockatoos and Sparrows in perfect harmony—-bliss.

Josh and Ralphie

Housesitting near the Sea is an added joy for me—a beach house!

Josh and Ralphie, two gorgeous, excited souls. Josh, a Schnauzer, and Ralphie, a Maremma, I arrived after dark quite late to a hidden key location, and much excitement from the Pooches was met with the key not wanting to open the door. They looked at me and I looked at them. They key jiggled, wiggled and ground in the lock to no avail. They were as frustrated as I was we couldn't get in. They pranced back and forth and I could intuitively hear their minds-chatter and see their facial expressions change from excitement to disgust. After help from a neighbour at an ungodly hour, the weeks following with great fun on beach walks, blissful facial expressions, and wirey-whisker-mouths receiving tasty treats.

Lovely Judy

Judy was a Dalmatian Coach dog with an elegant stance and Trott with her pristine black and white spotted coat. She was the family's baby; I'd have to wash her face with a cloth after her meals, she enjoyed parties and was the life of the party in fact. I minded Judy many times over many years; she would walk around in circles when they left and be there standing at the gate when they returned. Once, she sat with me in the backseat of the owner's car all the way from Victoria to Noosa for the annual holiday—about 2,000 km.

One of the additional pleasures of housesitting is free time. Most cats, dogs, birds, any unusual pets, gardens, antiques, and the houses themselves don't require 24/7 attention—allowing me the space to have personal time, to socialize, and to enjoy life—-a life of choice.

I have always enjoyed writing, and poetry, and writing little stories, so when the pets have settled down, I can get out my pen and paper.

Wherever you are, congratulations on a life well lived, you don't have to be afraid, just keep going. Have the courage to be mindful of your thoughts and channel them in a direction that is self-supporting—When your words are true and kind, they can change the world.

Take a look at yourself in the mirror and ask yourself, "Are you ready for my new story to begin?"

I leave you with a favorite saying of mine by Paul Solomon:

"I believe you came into the world to accomplish something, and that something you came to accomplish is not small or insignificant, that's not worthy of you. You came here to make a major contribution to life on this planet."
~ Paul Solomon, 1973. The Fellowship of The Inner Light, Paul Solomon Foundation.

About the Author

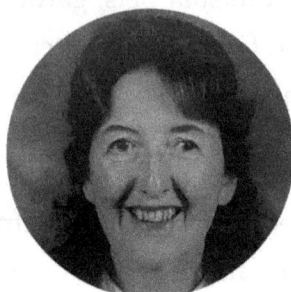

Marie Elson—Creator, Author, Housesitter, and Energy Wizard.

Marie realized one of her dreams to be a published Author, and now International bestselling author twice over. She resides on the Mornington Penninsula, Australia, and has traveled internationally exploring the globe and working in varied professions, travelling for adventure over the past 60 years. Her love for housesitting took her all over Australia, and now a proud Mother, Grandmother and Great-Grandmother.

If you don't see her in quiet meditation or walking over her Monet's Bridge, you will find her pruning her Roses, or making Plum Jam.

Mail: Marie Elson, % The Village Glen Residences. Capel Sound, Victoria, 3940, Australia.

-᷇W᷃W᷇→

Natalie and Isabella Fitzgerald

God isn't asking you to figure it out; he's asking you to trust that he already has.

Dreams Do Come True

It's not the morning dew that gathers on each blade of grass with the light being captured in each magical droplet, nor is it the orange and pink skies of brilliant country sunsets over the cow paddocks while hearing those last clucks from the chickens as they roost. As we sit and stare into the backyard crackling campfire at the end of a quiet weekend, it's the realization of long-held dreams that fill our hearts with joy. With 'Great Southern Land' by the band Icehouse playing in the background, our first YouTube video, titled *Our Little Patch of Paradise - on our Youtube chanel 'Our Family Farm, Gargett'*, goes live. It embodies the introduction to a beautiful story of what seems to be a new farm life but this story has only just begun.

Hi, I'm Natalie Fitzgerald, Wife, Mother, Business Owner, Youtuber, Farmer, and Author. Growing up I was always a little embarrassed by my middle name, Joy, I felt it was very old-fashioned, but I now believe this one word encapsulates my very essence. I aim to find it in everything I do, see and say to those around me. I have always had faith in god, felt spiritually attuned and if I'm honest... I've always been hopelessly optimistic about everything. I love nothing more than weekends spent at home pottering around doing odd jobs, reading a good crime novel in the bath or simply spending time cooking with my family.

Hi, I'm Isabella Fitsgerald, the co-author of this chapter and daughter of Natalie and Craig Fitzgerald. Student, Farmer, Author, Poet, Artist, Empath, and about to head into high school. I'm excited to publish some of my poetry (way out of my comfort zone of sharing my work). I love to read in general and am on a continual journey for discovery. I love Minecraft and online gaming, sharing my time with family. I feel that my independence has become me, and I love to do most things myself—like cooking my lunches and snacks. My favorite passions are writing, drawing, and playing games with Dad. Writing about whatever comes to mind at the time expresses my current mood and feelings, and I love everything horror and fantasy— I love both the escape and adventure of it all.

Many years ago, a mini-life audit had us figuring out where we stand on different areas of life: Health, Finances, Relationships, Career, Homelife, and Free Time. This pointed us toward an alternative, sustainable, high-quality life raising our daughter in paradise.

What is your paradise?

Our little patch of paradise came in the form of a small farm located 45 minutes outside Mackay, Queensland. Its long dirt driveway guides us past five fat Brangus cows grazing in lush green paddocks, and a white stone country cottage with its wide wrap-around veranda welcomes our arrival home. Our farm was going to allow us to achieve our dreams: becoming self-sufficient farmers with fruit trees, vegetable gardens, and meat from our cattle. We'd see our lives would slow down, creating a greater work-life balance, we'd get back in touch with each other and work together for the benefit of the farm.

"I like the farm

It's a lot different than life in town.

Many things seem to slow down,

And the more I spend out here -

The more everything seems more calm.

And THIS in now the place I hold very dear" —Isabella Fitzgerald

> *Stop stressing; I will get you through this.*
> ~ God

Our World is Rocked Again

What challenges make the most significant impact on your life?

It's no surprise that a cancer diagnosis in 2013 at the age of 30 was an incredibly difficult obstacle to overcome but with the help of modern medicine, I went into remission eight months later. So, you can only imagine our disbelief in the middle of moving, painting, unpacking, fixing chicken coops, acquiring livestock, and settling in came a second cancer diagnosis—a metastatic development from my first cancer over ten years earlier.

But this time, my doctors and their modern medicine could only hope to delay the inevitable. All of a sudden, I lost complete sight of the future. Our dreams of a simple life on the farm together, harvesting vegetables, drinking a morning coffee on the veranda with the view of the mountains, had vanished. My faith and ever-optimistic personality certainly wavered in those first couple of days until an incredible friend shared a podcast with Craig and I about the body's ability to achieve what the mind believes. Together, Craig and I decided to reject the doctor's diagnosis and their time frames and investigate alternative treatment options in addition to Western medicines.

it hurt. more than many. nothing i could have done. i can not do anything. nothing.~ Isabella Fitzgerald

During the first month, I began a tablet form of chemotherapy, drastically changed my diet, started bio-resonance therapy, and worked with a homeopath to boost my immune system. And after 6 weeks, the cancer count indicated a reduction by 100 points and my liver enzymes had improved dramatically. I also spent a lot of time rewriting my internal dialogue as discussed in the podcast, instructing my immune system "to locate and eliminate all cancer cells from my body right now." I believe that verbalising and visualizing my immune system fighting back against the cancer cells can only help in my recovery. I also spent a lot of time speaking to God about his plans for me, and I decided to unload the burden onto his shoulders. I can't do it by myself.

My rule of wellness is: The body achieves what the mind believes.

Living this life

We all noticed a massive shift with this recent diagnosis, and it's changed our family-run and owned Seafood business to its core––making immediate changes for us all personally. We, Craig, Myself, Bella, Mum, and Dad are making decisions for a better work/life balance and implementing changes; it is what we need for all our health, and we are gaining control of our happiness and health –strengthening relationships, living in the moment, living IN each day, LIVING daily/not just existing, surviving or going through the motions, doing things you want to do now, saying things now, creating experiences for Bella.

On Bella's last day of primary school in 2023, Craig dressed up in a Banana costume and arrived at the school in perfect timing when Bella emerged from her classroom. Her face flushes as she freezes, then lets out," Aw, Mum and Dad!!!!" as she tries to take off, no doubt to disappear under a rock; we are creating positive memories, photos, and videos that will be around for a long after we all are gone, I can imagine her showing her own children and grandchildren.

It is so important to continue living; our conversations aren't about cancer, my treatments or upcoming appointments, it's now just there in the background. We're living life to its fullest, putting up the Christmas tree and baking a gingerbread house, we're having adventures at our local waterway, this is a blissful place we go regularly to recharge. Not even a 5 min Buggy ride from the front gate through Sugar Cane paddocks, driving along the dirt road, the magnificent green valley parallels one of the creeks, and across the creek lies a rainforest where it is 5 deg cooler, smelling the fresh rainforest smell on the buggy is intoxicating. The refreshingly cool water of the stream tickles in parts and flows in others, but not freezing; we sit in it, walking along it and collecting the flat river rocks, skimming the stones over the pools of clear water, one of those places you can imagine recording the sounds; birds and animals and the water trickling sounds. We are recharging, cleansing, and connecting. Bella is a collector—a wonderful collection of river rocks now exists inside our home.

Isabellas' WOW moments: Live life to the fullest, whatever that looks like for you, your age, and your situation. Talking to her therapist and learning about 'the self' and that Darkness is not an affliction, but something to be honored (Poem below)

We are now enjoying the simple things in life, I inspect the growth of my zucchini plants, Bella oversees the hatching of the new little chicks and writes about her adventures, and Craig monitors the farm's fence lines. Our buggy takes the weekly Garbage bins down our long gravel driveway. The new habits we have formed are so far removed from city life and relationships with cows and chickens. Our cows are like dogs and when called, will run to us licking their lips in hopes of buckets of molasses. We bring vegetables scrapes home from the seafood cafe, and hand-feed the chickens and collect their eggs daily. I'm now pleased to be known as Mother-Hen, after we hand raised a new chick which was rejected by its mother. As I move about the house, the little chick follows me from room to room; if she loses me, she calls me with a distressed loud chirp. "Chubbs!" Bella named her due to her impressive fluffy feathers. "Mum, YUK, Chubbs pooed on the floor again," Bella yells, having stepped in the poop on the kitchen tiles.

Stay tuned for the upcoming publishing of our first children's book,' The Very Chirpy Chicken' that Bella and I are creating. Sharing the tiny miracles of life, miracles that occur on a farm that no one would know about less you do live on a farm. Our chickens have become a great source of hilarity, joy, and energy, a magnificent thing we want to share with the world.

God certainly had a plan for us and I feel like the farm came along at the right time, and is somehow a vital component of my healing. In the time we've lived here, Craig and I have developed an immense connection to the land and the joy it brings us every day is enormous. I believe the health of the farm and its animals is linked to my health, and this strengthens our resolve to be the best custodians of this farm.

Our plans to heal the land are twofold: as we heal the land, we're healing ourselves.

I feel a mirroring to be detoxifying the land and creating a magical environment for all creatures who live here; the weeding of the farm is a way of letting go (I feel the little toxic cells in my body being weeded out, too). Slashing and clearing the back paddocks of weeds, will allow an abundance of grass for the cows to eat, (clearing out everything inside me, creating a nourishing space for new cells to grow). Introducing manure and the chicken poop back into the land, composting, and creating our own fertilizer from fish frames (introducing support for my body from varied nourishments), partaking in carbon burns we burn off and pick up the ash and then put back into the ground, the embodiment of replenishing. Replacing all things lacking from my body and lacking from the farm, we are giving it new life – introducing love into each situation. The breath of the earth and my breath are flowing–the connection with the place. *Our little patch of paradise.*

Emotions sometimes run high, but love is always brought into every situation. Love is the dominant emotion that runs my life. You are only one decision away from a good mood and Paradise. Things happening in our lives, we don't understand, maybe it's God's plan we also cant see, don't understand, and just have to trust it. Some days when I'm feeling less than optimistic, simply spending time outside on the fresh green grass, asking for God's assistance, thinking about my family and friends, and all the reasons I have to fight, remind me to firm up my resolve.

Isabellas' new rule of wellness: Don't keep things bottled up inside yourself....as the results will literally explode. Telling others, "I'm so proud of you," is the magic behind everyone's self-confidence and self-love.

God has placed us on this land with this diagnosis for a reason, and I feel like by exploring mentally, spiritually, and physically we're doing what we're supposed to be doing. We're healing the land and ourselves, and along the way, we might find the reason that it was orchestrated to be so, but maybe we won't. Maybe it's just part of the journey and the life we were set to lead. Yes, this is the situation, I can be me. I feel the farm is also healing Craig and Isabella, I didn't know we all needed healing; it's a healing collective. And I feel we all need a metaphorical farm. Maybe this is the message I've lost all these past years— heal myself. I do hope everyone finds their own "farm," …not property, or a place, maybe a hobby, or anything that gives you time and space to not only be you but to heal.

My other New Rule for Wellness: Speak to every cell in your body and trust. Feel the healing connection to the land around you and express the twofold energy—heal and heal in return.

Isabella has one wish to impact the world—it's OK to heal and feel vulnerable.

Stop stressing, i will get you through this.
~ God

The Darkness of Night
by Isabella Fitzgerald

Filling some with fright
Minimal natural light,
The Darkness of Night.

Nocturnal creatures lurking
Dark waters murky,
The Darkness of Night.

People sleeping
People weeping,
The Darkness of Night.

Those who are traveling
Glancing at animals scavenging,
The Darkness of Night.

The sky blackening
Stars unveiling,
The Darkness of Night.

Mist rolling into the plain of green
Only darkness to be seen,
The Darkness of Night.

Sleeping tonight is challenging
So intense I'm imagining,
The Darkness of Night

About the Author

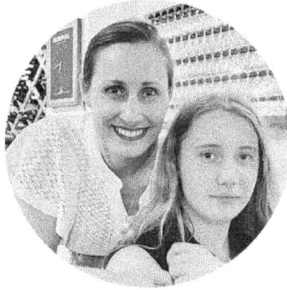

Natalie and Isabella Fitzgerald; Mother and Daughter team, living and loving life on their farm in Gargett, Far North Queensland, with Father and Husband Craig, and many fur-baby family members, Bovine neighbors, and years of magnificent sunsets.

You will find Nataie and Isabella in the farm kitchen creating magnificent aromas cooking up a storm, and if Natalie is not creating culinary magic, you will find her in her garden. She loves creating sweet delights with Isabella and enjoying them on the porch in the late afternoons.

Isabella will be with 'Chubb's' and her feathers friend's family — sorting out the pecking order in the chicken coop collecting their eggs, and totally in her element when the hens fight to sit on her shoulder.

Email: natalie.fitzgerald@bigpond.com
YouTube: Our Family Farm Gargett

-/\/\/\→

Sharon Grant

Dear Friend

In that moment you feel empty and in despair,
No matter how busy my life; I'm always there.
I too feel those moments I'm lost and alone,
The direction of tomorrow; seems so unknown,
But you take a breath and in that foggy moment your family
pays a glimpse,
And a little strength you gain from all the past you've shared
together since.
The weather will settle and tomorrow will clear,
and those fears so strong yesterday, a little less near.
Something makes you smile, and those memories will soon fade,
Each day from now your strength will grow, self-punishment
you've paid,
So Dear Friend please know, my offer of time is surely true,
And for someone whose so special, I'm always there for you...

New Leaf

It found us really, where the stars align and the degrees just right, is a Little Farm in the lower Hunter Valley.

Slowly entering the road, the creek follows alongside a mass of cornflower blue water lilies in bloom, surrounded by hills abundant with sandstone rocks.

I was not quite 50, and the world wasn't the one we'd known.

Melbourne had restricted us beyond ok, and it didn't feel like home anymore apart from our friends.

Living in the growth corridor, the surrounding suburbs becoming so congested; made driving anywhere an unpleasant frustration.

Our beautiful property was so hard to leave, and it took months to find something suitable, and we never imagined we'd move so far.

Down the very bumpy road, we drove wondering if we could manage to do this daily?

We found the old gate entry. and the pig sign attached by the entrance. A rusty pig on the black letter box and knew we were here.

We stayed the night in a nearby town half an hour away to return in the morning to take it in and walk amongst the forest, with a plan to make it ours.

It happened so quickly that we sold within five days, and we were packed and gone in 30. Making our way in our old motorhome, Utes and two trailers loaded, my daughter and I with the float, her pony and nine chickens.

15 hours it took with fuel stops, a puncture, regular pony rests, keeping the water up to the chickens. We arrived late; after two traffic camera fines, and kindly three eggs laid by the girls.

Further than we had expected with a few back steps, but the right foundation to begin again.

Apart from the chooks, we brought fruit trees and seeds to start a little orchard and grow a few veggies of course all that would take time, but we aimed to be as organic as possible.

Gardening is better than therapy.

My Journey to Me

I met my future husband when I was 18, he was handsome, very interesting, and made me laugh, but dating someone I worked with. I didn't know then that he would later change my life, and together we would be an awesome team.

I grew up in the beautiful seaside town of Mornington with my amazing parents. Brought up to take my shoes off and always bring a plate of food when visiting. Respect your elders and always lend a hand.

Going along as the average young adult, I had done my secretarial diploma back when shorthand was taught, switchboards used, and a smile in your voice welcomed customers to business. Publisher and excel a fitting structure to begin a journey of administration and supporting backbone to a multitude of companies.

Goal-focused working in real estate, modeling on a minor scale for Myers, and Laura Ashley, teaching deportment and confidence to 2-16yr olds.

Then going overseas with my partner for a few months and coming home to get married.

Lasting only a couple of years, I learnt that if the foundations not strong enough in a relationship, you will not survive life's struggles.

I had a marvelous paying job and a boss who saw my potential that I respected, the lady in the office however wanted me out, going to great lengths to make it uncomfortable. Intimidated by my age and modern technology. With struggles in my job and marriage, it all came crashing down, I was failing myself. I went into my shell; shaking in the bath, wanting to just disappear. With enough sick leave and holiday pay, I finished work. I was low like I had never known.

Turning to Nature

I re- met my future husband when I was 23 through a friend and learned about his business in organics and growing of natural food. We spoke all night about everything; I said you don't want to get mixed up with me, my life is a mess, and he said sort it out and I will wait.

I got a job running an office for a kind gentleman with cancer selling farm supplies at his property. Helping my partner and friends at their organic farm run production, packaging the fruits etc. I designed a logo, brochure, and market stall my partner built. We would package extra products on the side with my parents' help.

After a while went our own way, having different views on the business direction we moved to Gembrook. Buying an old caravan, setting up a simple life off the grid amongst the forest.

We had two beautiful children, not without the normal difficulties first deciding when to have them and us both being ready. After a long and painful birth, we shared the arrival of our wonderful son.

Three years later blessed with our gorgeous daughter, brought on early to avoid a similar situation. I got my little cappuccino queen.

A relocatable home now and the want to build, juggled work and kids. My husband saw a need in the packaging industry, so a small group of us decided to start a business in manufacturing.

We struggled to get it going all working hard, painting floors, building internal structures, and kept moving forward anyway we could. Working on the side to keep putting in, my parents helping with the children. We would sleep between their house and the factory. We all sold what we could keeping things going, even an overdraught against my parent's house. It was just us initially packaging with lots of 2nd hand parts, my husband and brother installed to get us going. It was a real team effort. Finally getting our first cheque, we hired staff, good people, and hard working. Hired another factory and packaged there too just to keep them in a job.

Then things took a real back step we never saw coming and didn't want to face. My niece at age 12 was diagnosed with brain cancer.

It was tough, everyone rallied we did what we could, it was a 4 ½ year emotional battle. It affected us all so much, but we had to keep going we had other children to support and staff to keep in jobs and so much invested we could not give up. We carried things amongst us, for another 4 ½ years. Ten years in total our business had grown to 5 factories and 67 staff, we were exhausted but with a good team of people sold our business with an outcome that left us all more than comfortable. We did not celebrate as we hoped, too much had happened, and we have all gone our separate ways. The balance of life in this is the extreme success and the extreme loss to match. Money does not bring happiness.

You cannot make the scars in your life disappear, but you can change the way you view them.

Healing and forgiving myself took time to truly investigate the depths of the person in the mirror where I saw my grandmother, mother, self, niece, and daughter. Their lessons learned and taught, similarities, every wrinkle gained from smiles and stresses. Your daughter's beauty, youth, and struggles, the strength to find herself, and the respect for the women that have gone the journey before her. The voyage up till now has made me a more gracious person. I like who I am becoming, finding gratitude in each day and the strength to be the best version of myself.

Creating a new dream and focusing on that together, the movie of your life you hope and continue to strive for, and whatever does not make sense today will find its place tomorrow.

Take time to care for others and be kind, encourage where you can. I was fortunate enough to give back and care for someone who was a big part of my life as a child. She too had cancer, and I was blessed to share one day a week with her, never reminding her of her illness just enjoying one another's company. There is nothing more rewarding than to have someone allow you to help them when they are at their most vulnerable. To be trusted like that is so very precious.

I am far from a perfect person, wife, or mother, or even friend, but I am learning all the time and listening is the biggest lesson, or you miss so much. Funnily enough, as we get older, we forget what we want to say and quite often speak over each other, not to be more important just to say things while we remember. Baby brain was one thing, but menopause is another.

I could say I am just a mum, but my mother would pull me up on that because as a mother we are so much more, never to be undervalued. (Plumber, cook, nurse, taxi driver, housekeeper, social worker, painter, and gardener etc).

A selected few, I share a place at my table of Camelot where we are all equal.

I can be strong in my own way, some days more than others, but so much stronger with the people that surround me, my mentors, and dear friends. Each giving me knowledge, strength, guidance of various kinds. Healthier for their love, kindness and support and them from mine. Sneaking time where we can to share a hug, coffee, or tea and a good D and M.

Solving the world's problems, laughing, and crying together and find the time is never long enough, feeling better for sharing when ending a call. We're so blessed to have such amazing people to share our journey; they are such a cherished part of our family's life.

My darling friend said to me "What are you doing today that your future self will be thank you for?" How beautiful is she, we have known each other 37yrs and a smile always finds my face when I think of her.

Better Together

My husband is my rock, he makes me question myself, my strongest motivator, driving me to be the best version of myself. Knowing that whatever we are doing we are part of an effective team, with our own journey on the same path. I chose him at the beginning and ending of each day. My husband calls me Pepper like in Ironman, and he Starky. We are a driving force, each driving the other if the other is down, staying focused on our goals in business, home, and family. Staying connected with all life throws at you, growing children, appreciating each other after an empty nest.

The biggest lessons I have learnt from him and always share are "Make a movie make it happen!" "You can only have what you see for yourself."

My parents are two of the most kind and caring people I know, my biggest comfort, always listening and wanting the best for me. I love them dearly and can never do enough for their support.

My children have taught me so much. Not to micromanage, allow them to find their paths. Taught me to chill, worry less and enjoy every moment we can. Grateful I always took them out of school as a treat on their birthday.

Knowing that they are the only two people to know my heart from the inside.

Functions and renovations are my passion- Organising is in my blood, coming from a family of builders, caterers and creative mother means events have come naturally. Creating lots of business dinners, Christmas functions for staff and our families to the perfect kids themed party and 80ths at the Eureka Towers and Rippon Lea. Inspired by making someone's day special or occasion perfect for them. If it allows someone to sparkle, then it is worth the effort. Hoping to incorporate that now with our beautiful surrounds, my Tiny Houses, organic produce, and weddings in our little hidden paradise.

Breaking the circle to Health

For too long it was almost three-monthly rinse and repeat of weight up, weight down, achieve, achieve, achieve then crash and cry, find the couch with your much needed friends nurofen, ice and heat pack, looking a sorry site yet again. Why do I keep repeating this? Is it all I know, or can I finally find a new path and realise this is not working. Finally voiced it to me and then to him. I live my life alongside yours, but I must travel it in my own lane. After children and with menopause, need to do what works for me. With my new attitude I chose with my naturopath to remove foods that inflame my body, to eat organically, exercise and stress less.

You cannot heal or lift yourself up, until you can unconditionally forgive your own faults, misunderstandings, and ignorance's then the true lessons of life may be offered.

What works for me

A routine of Apple cider Vinegar, lemon, and honey to start each day, stretch my body like my father taught me and he still does at 82 every morning. Finish will a salute of the sun as it feels so grounding to begin a day with.

Being off the grid and working towards a sustainable life in organic surroundings and respecting nature. When life seems overwhelming; and should haves, would haves, could haves sneak upon you. I now take a different approach; apart from lists and take time to relax and centre myself. Is there a rush to do any of it? Contemplate and find a pace that is achievable of a good day's effort, allowing me to enjoy each thing on my list, from making meals to pulling weeds so that I don't dread to go back to these things the next time they need tending rather than tackling. Balance the day with a little bit of everything not to feel weighed down, but the continuation of achievement always finding time throughout the day for my dog. Just get started from anywhere or any corner and before you know it, it has been done. *Don't look at the mountain ahead but look just beyond your feet and the top is closer than you realise!* Take the focus off the size and make it about each step. Of course, both these things are better with the company, taking turns with the baton and being gentle on yourself. Looking towards expanding our eatable garden and harvesting the vegies and fruit and preparing and sharing it with family and friends. I have learnt to install irrigation, make bread, pasta and preserve food. Aiming to try my hand in growing fish, and yabbies for dad to enjoy homemade fish n chips.

Supporting my husband in our new business in medicinal cannabis, in the hope to help people in the balance of health and self.

Getting off Facebook (Hubby calls the mirror in the budgie cage) unless it's for business. Keeping off phones and connecting to the world, it has so much to offer and share as do you, especially through a hug, touch and smile that's so important.

When the house is yours find time for date night, enjoy nibbles, a glass of wine and each other, taking turns for a massage, and hot tub.

The night sky hear can touch your soul..

Listening to my podcast and not just music, means I learn alot. Then when I have time, I put the roof down and connect with the world around. Shake off the sillies dancing around the lounge room with the music up loud, making homemade pizza with the family.

Be present- I find healing in my garden, listening to the birds, take time to feel the breeze, talk to the angel's, planting seeds and nurturing myself in breath and in the pleasure of a simple moment.

Don't wait for someone to tell you you're dying before you truly embrace life and see the true beauty in the world.

Find sunsets in everyday moments to cherish.

We start each day on our beautiful farm in the valley with the view through the wide glass windows and invite the morning in slowly to the rise of the sun, as the sounds of the rooster crowing confirms it's start.

The dogs nose rests upon the bedside and we sit up and allow ourselves to wake, she hops up and awaits her traditional belly rub and early morning spoilers.

In the orchard you can see the wallaby mother's gather with babies in and out of pouches grazing in the safety of the farmyard fences.

The dew from the morning begins to steam from the grass with each touch of the sun.

Making time with the soil, breeze, and sun with the chickens at my feet, as I care for the trees I have planted to connect with this wonderful earth.

Preparing the tiny houses in the hope to create a special moment for those that chose to stay and embrace this place and its beauty too.

Finding the days end as the temperature drops and the Kookaburras serenade us with their echoing voices, the fog sets in, the sun goes down and the blanket lays again over our Little Valley Farm.

Remembering to fall asleep with your dream and wake up with a purpose.

About the Author

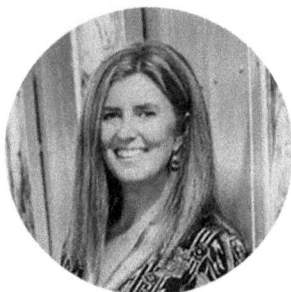

Sharon Grant; "Je suis comme je suis" (I am what I am). She is Women, Wife, Mother, Daughter, Friend, Function Co-ordinator, Farmer, Housewife...and more. She doesn't believe success to just be in business or the certificates held, but that person's contribution of to the world, and to be the best versions of ourselves with kindness and purpose.

Sharon, with nearly 50 years of calling Melbourne home, now plants new roots amongst the Lower Hunter Valley in NSW. Renovations and functions her passion, but her garden and connection to nature are her haven for self-growth, now inviting people to share and stay amongst it's beauty and just be.

Creating this chapter content has been very fulfilling, with self-reflection and the opportunity to be able to write and bring my lessons to the world.

Email: Lillies and Limestone Tiny Houses: sharon@asj.net.au

-ᴡᴡᴡ→

Tia-Kalinya

SHE is Magick™

As I sit down a day overdue for this final submission, I'm reminded that my story often unfolds under the weight of pressure—a theme that echoes throughout my life. Much like a diamond forged in the crucible of darkness, it's during these moments of intense strain that I come alive, radiating light through the multifaceted facets of my being. Before delving into my transformation, let's rewind to a time when my life was a canvas painted with different hues of emotion and challenge. It's a journey marked by the struggles I faced—the sleepless nights, the unfulfilled desires, and the relationships that shaped but didn't define me. My turning point, the crucible of change, awaited, and when it arrived, it set me on a path of profound self-discovery.

Fast forward to the present, where the echoes of transformation resonate. The metamorphosis didn't come without its challenges, but the rewards have been profound. My life has evolved, and I stand amidst three significant benefits—each a testament to the power of change. The landscape of my relationships has transformed, reflecting the newfound strength within. I've achieved goals that once seemed insurmountable, mirroring the aspirations many of my clients harbor.

Now, as I contemplate the future, a vision for impact begins to take shape. Leading from the heart, I envision a ripple effect of positive change—one that extends beyond personal victories to touch the lives of others. SHE is Magick™, forged in the crucible of my experiences, become a guiding light for those seeking transformation. The journey ahead holds the promise of greater impact as I aspire to share the gifts gained during this transformative odyssey with the ordinary world, inspiring others to embark on their own path of self-discovery.

In the quiet corners of my ordinary world, the tapestry of my journey began to unfold, woven with threads of challenge, yearning, and the quest for self-discovery. The ordinary world, seemingly unremarkable to an outsider, held the silent echoes of my aspirations and struggles, the prelude to a transformative odyssey.

Growing up, I found myself navigating a maze of challenges that cast shadows on my path to belonging, trust, and love. The roots of my transformation can be traced back to these formative years—a time when I yearned for connection but stumbled upon the jagged terrain of isolation. It was an era of uncertainty, where the mirror reflected a version of myself yearning for validation, acceptance, and a sense of purpose.

Amidst the ordinary backdrop of school days and familial interactions, the seeds of resilience were sown. The early chapters of my life unfolded against a canvas painted with the hues of self-discovery, as I grappled with the fundamental human desires to be seen, heard, and valued. The mirror of adolescence reflected not just physical changes but also the evolving contours of my identity—a complex mosaic of dreams, fears, and latent potential.

The catalyst for my transformation lay dormant within the mundane moments, waiting for the right alignment of circumstances to awaken its power. It was unnecessary to provide a chronological overview of every chapter in my life; instead, I offer you a snapshot of a key starting point, a crossroads where the ordinary world met the extraordinary potential within.

This starting point, seemingly unassuming, marked the genesis of my journey toward self-discovery. It was a call to adventure, an invitation to embark on a path that would redefine my understanding of self, purpose, and the interconnectedness of all things. Little did I know that the ordinary world was merely the cocoon from which the butterfly of transformation would emerge, spreading its wings to explore the vast landscapes of possibility and purpose.

As I invite you into the corridors of my ordinary world, I encourage you to reflect on your own starting point—the moments that became the ink with which your life's narrative began. It is within these seemingly commonplace moments that the extraordinary often takes root, waiting for the opportune moment to unfurl its wings and soar into the realm of possibility.

***

In the symphony of life, the crescendo of change echoed in the aftermath of an unexpected discord—my broken back. Lying immobilised, contemplating the uncertain future that hung in the balance between surgery and the dreams I once held dear, I found myself at a crossroads. It was a moment of vulnerability, a plea to the universe for respite, a break from the relentless challenges that had defined my recent past.

In the stillness of recovery, a digital sanctuary emerged—a virtual refuge offering an eclectic blend of spiritual work, meditation, neurobiology hacking, business coaching, and entrepreneurship. This online community became the catalyst for my Call to Adventure, the gateway to a transformative journey that transcended the confines of my comfort zone. What began as a quest for solace evolved into a multidimensional exploration of self-discovery.

The initial immersion into this virtual realm became a daily ritual, marked by master classes, webinars, and transformative practices that stretched from sunrise to sunset. It was within this digital cocoon that the alchemy of change commenced, reshaping the contours of my perception and guiding me towards a new path.

The backdrop to this transformation was my life in Indonesia, where I had spent months immersed in ocean conservation for tourism during my final year of university in my 30s. The collision of diverse cultures elicited a range of emotions—thrill, heartbreak, humility, and unbridled joy. Plans to build a career overseas crumbled with the fracture in my back, a week before Christmas, precisely when my final assessments were due to complete my bachelor's degree. The dreams I had nurtured seemed to disintegrate, leaving me with a singular focus on finishing my degree, oblivious to the deeper currents of transformation swirling beneath the surface.

The path back to becoming a medicine woman mirrored the shamanic concept of a thousand cuts—I was poked, prodded, gently held, and encouraged to walk my spirit path. Yet, I remained oblivious to the signs, the cosmic whispers urging me to embrace my true calling. It wasn't until the echoes of those whispers became impossible to ignore that I embarked on the transformative journey laid before me. The ordinary world, marked by the constraints of academia and the shattered dreams of a life overseas, yielded to the extraordinary possibilities that awaited in the realm of spiritual awakening.

***

In the embrace of recovery, my sanctuary shifted to the serenity of home along the banks of the Clarence River, where my father and his partner played the role of compassionate architects of my revival. Their inspiration, encouragement, love, and unwavering support became the scaffolding upon which I rebuilt my life. This pivotal stage, akin to Crossing the Threshold, saw me standing at the gateway of transformation, ready and committed to a journey with no turning back.

The resounding affirmation from neurosurgeons, granting me the all-clear to resume life's adventures without surgery, ignited a spark within. Although scuba and horseback riding lay on a distant horizon, the freedom from immediate medical concerns beckoned me back to the northern rivers, NSW—the lush landscape of my roots. Here, within the embrace of ancestral lands, I immersed myself in a tapestry of spiritual experiences— spirit fests, women's song, plant medicine ceremonies, and solstice celebrations. It was a return to the heart of the medicine woman and the medicine people, guided by the traditional custodians of the land.

Barefoot, raw, and physically broken, I navigated each day as a conscious step forward. Every sunrise became a testament to resilience, as I waded through the currents of pain, loneliness, loss, isolation, and lingering terror. The path was arduous, but with each gentle and deliberate step, the transformation unfolded.

In this crucible, I rediscovered the essence of my authentic self, a little girl within me yearning for protection and love—an inner companion neglected for far too long. The journey toward healing became a collaborative effort as the wounded parts of me found solace and strength in each other. Together, we ventured into the realms of self-discovery, exploring the scars and vulnerabilities that shaped our narrative.

Returning to the roots of my being allowed me not only to mend the fractures within but also to extend a helping hand to others on their healing odysseys. It's through this shared experience that the authentic healer within me emerged—a conduit for empathy, understanding, and genuine connection. The Crossing of the Threshold marked not just the commencement of my personal transformation but also the genesis of a purposeful journey toward guiding others through their own passages of healing and self-discovery.

***

As I ventured further into the labyrinth of my transformation, roadblocks emerged as stern tests of strength and willpower. Among the myriad challenges, one of the most formidable was the quest for stable accommodation—a necessity that loomed large in the absence of a steady income. For years, my reliance on welfare became a lifeline as I invested in my own healing journey.

The landscape of my life during this period resembled a patchwork quilt of impermanence, where couch surfing, house sitting, and camping became not just occasional adventures but prominent features of my daily existence. The quest for a stable haven was arduous, as each day presented a new puzzle to solve, a new place to adapt to, and a new challenge to overcome.

In the crucible of uncertainty, a turning point materialised in the form of a significant ally—my new partner. Their arrival on the scene was nothing short of providential, offering not only emotional support but also becoming a pivotal force in creating a stable foundation. Together, we dismantled the barriers that stood between me and a secure dwelling, reshaping the narrative of my transient existence.

This period, marked by tests and trials, also revealed the resilience inherent in the human spirit. The foes I faced were not external adversaries but the internal demons of doubt, insecurity, and the constant whispers of inadequacy. Each day became a battleground, where the rules of engagement were learned through a combination of grit, adaptability, and unwavering determination.

Amidst the trials, a mentor emerged not in the conventional sense but in the form of divine guidance—the subtle nudges from the universe, signaling that I was on the right path. The moments of clarity were like beacons in the darkness, illuminating the way forward. It was in these instances of synchronicity, where the threads of my journey wove seamlessly with the cosmic fabric, that I found reassurance that I was not alone.

The challenges, once formidable foes, transformed into steppingstones—each one propelling me forward on the journey toward self-discovery and healing. It was a metamorphosis of the spirit, a testament to the indomitable strength that surfaces when faced with adversity. Through the support of allies and the moments of divine guidance, the roadblocks became opportunities for growth, and the path forward began to unveil itself with newfound clarity.

**

As I transitioned back to Queensland and stepped into the role of a facilitator for the Red Tent, my journey as a practitioner took on a profound new dimension. It was within this vibrant community, guided by my mentor Jill and embraced by fellow kindred spirits, that I discovered another layer of my calling—the sister wound. Here, my narrative truly began to unfold as I committed myself to working with women, for women, to foster growth—a challenge that has become one of the most rewarding chapters of my life.

Accountability, resilience, adaptability—these became the cornerstones of my work. It meant choosing to overcome the barriers that held us back, confronting the limitations, and resisting the allure of regression into the 'safe place,' that comfortable haven where avoidance shields us from facing our actions and imperfections. True growth began when we collectively decided to shed the cocoon of comfort and step into the raw vulnerability of self-discovery.

Over the years, I have had the privilege of working with thousands of individuals, predominantly women. My mission has been to guide them in uncovering the layers that hinder personal growth, providing tools for transformation, teaching emotional regulation, and emphasising the importance of self-care and forgiveness—both for others and, most crucially, for ourselves.

My journey of impact has been enriched by diverse modalities and qualifications, ranging from somatic embodiment and naturopathy to various massage modalities, red tent circles, shamanic medicine, phenomenology, human behavioural science, and business foundations. Each qualification has served as a brushstroke in the tapestry of my capabilities, expanding the palette from which I draw to guide others toward their transformative potential.

A poignant letter from my mentor, Jill, encapsulates the essence of my journey: 'Tia is an observer; she watches from the edges and anticipates the needs of everyone in the room. Her lightning-speed movements, speech, and infectious laughter are coupled with an uncanny ability to intuit what's coming next and what's needed, showcasing a keen awareness. Her courage to 'own her shit' in the pursuit of becoming a better person is truly admirable. Tia possesses the gift of speaking her truth, even if it triggers the calmest among us, addressing what everyone is thinking, but few are courageous enough to vocalise. She stands as a sentinel of loyalty and trustworthiness, a person of strong integrity, honesty, and reliability. I would trust her with my life.'

In a recent exchange with my circle, a testament to the impact I've made emerged: 'A powerful woman who encompasses the goddesses in all their glory, always seeking the best in everyone to empower them through their journeys. Tia is moved to create a home for others, to encourage raw emotion and need.

'She is Magick. She is Tia-Kalinya.'

These words resonate as a reflection of the communal embrace, affirming that the impact stretches beyond individual transformations, creating a ripple effect that extends to the empowerment and communal upliftment of those around me.

***

As I traverse the realms of my transformative journey, the Return to the ordinary world takes shape through Ámëntì, a community dedicated to exploring the fifth dimension—a metaphysical realm that transcends the boundaries of the physical and delves into higher levels of consciousness. In the fifth dimension, unity and interconnectedness prevail, offering an opportunity for heightened awareness and a profound sense of cosmic calibration.

Christian Bernard's poignant quote serves as the guiding principle for Ámëntì, encapsulating the essence of carrying the whole of humanity forward as we progress individually. The community engages in cosmic calibration and tribal gatherings, aligning ancient primordial bodies with spiritual highways to connect with universal energy. It's a quest to step into the 'real' life, where we tap into a great universal power and unlock answers to our deepest questions, including the pursuit of happiness.

As a phenomenologist, I contribute to this quest by analysing and reflecting on the nature of human experience. Grounded in the belief that careful examination and reflection can unveil the essence of human experience, my work delves into the structure of consciousness, the role of embodiment in experience, and the profound impact of culture and society on our perceptions of the world.

The collaborator in this cosmic exploration, I dedicate my career to understanding the intricate tapestry of human experience. Drawing on disciplines such as philosophy, psychology, and anthropology, my research aims to shed new light on the structure of consciousness, the importance of embodiment in experience, and the ways culture shapes our perceptions. It's a trailblazing endeavour with the potential to transform our understanding of the human experience.

In the pursuit of greater impact, the SHE is Magick™ journey emerges as a beacon, guiding women through a nine-month transformative odyssey. Rooted in the archetypal wisdom of Carl Jung, Jean Shinoda Bolen, Maureen Murdock, Clarissa Pinkola Estés, and Marion Woodman, this journey unlocks somatic and intuitive wisdom, facilitating self-healing and liberation from daily stress.

Empowering women with practical tools and practices within the SHE is Magick™ curriculum, the journey promotes physical, mental, and emotional well-being. It is a commitment to creating a safe and transformative space where women can relax, rejuvenate, and allow their nervous systems to experience deep states of relaxation and restorative rest.

Embracing emotional regulating techniques, the SHE is Magick™ journey guides women on a path of stress reversal, enabling them to reclaim their natural state of aliveness, freedom, ecstasy, and grounded embodiment. The focus is on empowering women to skillfully regulate their emotions, embodying archetypal resilience and cultivating a harmonious connection between mind, body, and spirit.

Beyond the journey, the SHE is Magick™ initiative aims to build a global community of empowered and awakened women. This community, influenced by decades of expertise, fosters enduring connections that contribute to a network of transformation and empowerment across the globe. It's a vision that transcends individual healing, creating a ripple effect that touches the lives of women far beyond the confines of the transformative journey.

In essence, my vision for greater impact in the future is woven into the fabric of cosmic exploration, community empowerment, and transformative journeys. It is a commitment to unlocking the potential for healing, growth, and interconnectedness, reaching beyond the individual to contribute to the collective evolution of humanity.

About the Author

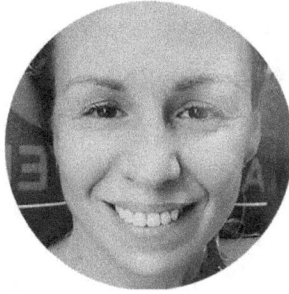

With over two decades in metaphysical and human sciences, Tia embarked on a transformative journey, blending communal living with academic ascent.

Born into a family rooted in transcendental meditation, herbal medicine, and mystic practices, Tia inherited a passion for transformative power. Relentlessly pursuing a bachelor's degree and earning numerous diplomas and certificates, they formed expertise through academic and practical channels.

Tia facilitates transformative spaces, advocating for humanity's innate ability to turn pain into faith. As a guide, they empower individuals on unique transformational journeys, prioritising resilience, adaptability, and bliss.

Tia's mission transcends personal growth, committing to global positive change by alchemizing challenges into opportunities. Join her on this odyssey where fear transforms into trust, paving the way for a harmonious Existence.

SHE is Magick™ * Tia-Kalinya * Phenomenologist

Email: Tia@SheisMagick.com
Website: https://www.SheisMagick.com
Facebook: https://www.facebook.com/AmentiOfficial

-⌁⟶

Dani Jasmine Middendorp

When we all existed as pure energy, the Higher Power said: "Do you want to go to Earth for a very, very short amount of time— like a blip of time, and experience all the emotions, fears, anxieties, joys, and gravity? Would you?"

YES, I certainly would!

Interesting, isn't it? As that pure energy, we want to experience different things; when we *are* experiencing different things now on earth as Beings, we want to know what ELSE is out there, what is up there higher than us? If there is *even* a higher us, and intrigued with all the answers to the Universe—we 'feel' there is something else, but we can't recall exactly.

We are always on a search or on a journey to find it.

Maybe it's time to experience our life as it currently is. Do the things, meet the people, travel, eat the foods, taste the emotions, feel them, float in the water, and feel the sensations—all Of it. Live consciously and just purely enjoy all that you are and have.

Simple.

My new rule for wellness: You focus on you, then you grow, you focus on s*it, then s*it grows.

My Mother sends me a card she has chosen for me most weeks, a lovely way to commence my day—and I love it so much, we did this when I was a small child, growing up, we did this as a kind of daily meditation and thought intention. As an older teenager, this became a guiding force in my life, and now, as an adult living and travelling elsewhere in the world, It's a reminder of a guiding energy, a direction to focus on.

I sit in my bed in Canada with the wilderness of the Cascade Mountains out my window with the brightness of the full Moon pouring in and landing on my bed covers. I look at the card Mum has sent me just now—It's her late afternoon in Australia, my bedtime after my late work shift. The card is the Ace of Gabriel from the Archangel POWER cards by Doreen Virtue and Radleigh Valentine, Hay House Publication Inc, 2005, reprint 2013. (Mum's favourite set she has had for Donkey's years), it depicts a woman with her wings spread afa; she holds a long golden trumpet set in what looks reminiscent of a German Village with a Mountainous backdrop.

The message reads:

'It's a time to take action when you are called to take up whatever activity motivates you the most, great chances to move forward in your life. A wonderful gift to accept new adventures and opportunities"...

I feel this card offers me permission to go forth with a sense of wonder, to enrich my soul and my soul's journey. Ultimately, that has brought me to Canada.

"...A gift of passion, opportunity, and inspiration. The chance to do something amazing! A sense of Wonder."

This very card holds great significance in my life. It was the very first card I had ever chosen out of this pack when Mum first acquired them—the image of the Winged girl I have had tattooed on my arm as it resonates with me and is so significant.

Certain things happen in your life that you can't find the meaning behind; maybe we aren't meant to 'find the meaning' at all, for some things seem senseless and unfair, some things are cruel and break your heart into a million pieces, some things bring you so much Joy and connection, and healing too. I've done so many things already in my 27 years on this Planet, but I felt something was lacking, and my 'experiencing' all these things. Mum one day, when I was feeling particularly low and down, said, "Remember all the stars you had in your eyes for your future so many years ago?" In that very instant, time stood still, I did remember. "What did you want to do with all your passion many years ago?" she continued.

"All I wanted to do was go to Canada, Mum!" I unintentionally yelled back through a haze of tears.

"Well, let's get you to Canada!" she beamed at me.

My gaze back wasn't a 'beam of sparkle' like she gave me. That instant was filled with the doom and gloom of the 'reality' of not being in a financial state to afford to go to Canada, not to mention starting life, a new adventure for a couple of years over there either. Millions of thoughts were racing through my head about how 'it wouldn't happen.' Well, Mum called me out on that also. "I'll make it happen, somehow, and you can meet the people, travel, eat the foods, taste the Canadian Vibe, feel the emotions, feel the countryside, float in the water, and feel the sensations!"

Somehow, it did happen, and now I'm here, adding to my Soul's journey. What is the path really like? Love, love lost, travel, many destinations, energy, learning, trust—and so much more. This spellbinds me, and in fact, you can read it even as a spiritual teaching; I feel the below prose says it all and is suggestive of clear and direct wisdom is revealed:

The soul's journey is a path of love,
A journey of light and grace,
A journey of surrender and trust,

A journey to the beloved's embrace.
The journey begins with a longing,
A yearning for the divine,
A thirst for the nectar of love,
A desire for the eternal shrine.
The journey leads through many lands,
Through deserts and mountains and seas,
Through valleys of darkness and light,
Through forests of joy and peace.
The journey is a test of faith,
A challenge to the heart and soul,
A journey of surrender and grace,
A journey to the beloved's goal.
~ Lal Shahbaz Qalandar

Lal Shahbaz Qalandar was a revered Sufi saint, poet, and musician who lived in the 12th century in what is now modern-day Pakistan. He preached a message of tolerance, inclusivity, and spiritual enlightenment, and his poetry and teachings continue to inspire people of diverse backgrounds and faiths. Love it.

Living in British Columbia far exceeds my expectations, and living in a little historic town that means a "valley of many streams" is heavenly. The town that has a church square and a church bell, with the city motto as " the green heart of the province". Magic. So idyllic.

There are endless things to do in Canada for a travel lover. It's a four-season playground, but the best thing... I've found love!

For years I saw myself hiking in the Canadian wilderness, Mum even envisioned me working as a Zoologist in a Wolf rescue park (I don't even know if Wolf rescue parks even exist!).

Each year, tourists flock to the Tundra and see Bears, Birds of Prey soar high in Banff National Park, and ohhhhhh the hot springs—one day for sure. Currently, I'm living in this historical village—reminiscent of the town from the TV show Gilmore Girls—Mum and I used to love watching it, and both said, 'I'd love to live there!' Well, I feel I am living there—-living my dream for sure. I can see myself snowshoeing; the snow has just begun to fall—like giant feathers falling gently from the sky, I never knew snowflakes could be so big. So blissful.

I feel I've always overthought things in general— overthinking– I love you so—overthinking—I won't let you go— overthinking—you break me—overthinking—you make me rise again.

I ask myself many questions: How can I surrender even more in this very moment and not bring in everything else I'm thinking about? Where am I called to use my voice right now? How can I infuse more self-love and compassion into my daily life?

Answer—I'm not entirely sure. I haven't figured it all out, but

I'm working on it, and I will share it with you. Maybe this is one way, in the amazing book, to share my voice with the world.

I feel it's essential to have clear, strong intentions–and desires, yet I'm still learning to detach from the outcome. No plan—No victory! It's time to set a series of 'motions' on the course and wait. It's time to surrender; I struggle with this, too. Let go of the wheel and trust. Mum reminds me of this often. Let trust turn into gratitude for what you still cannot see—but know it's coming—I love this. To action this: know this (so deeply that your soul vibrates): YOU ARE NOT ALONE. Your life has a purpose; the more you surrender, the more miracles will be produced.

My mantra is, "I surrender, I accept all that I cannot change, I release the outcome, and I joyfully trust the process."

I believe I have a soul script—your story matters—written so it can be spoken. Share your story, be brave, and speak your truth. Your voice is the catalyst for healing others; you never know ONE word may change them.

> *"If your compassion does not include yourself, it is incomplete."* ~ Buddha

CHOOSE ONE SELF-CARE ACTION TO DO TODAY:

- Set strong boundaries
- Meditate, listen to your heart, listen to music

- Refer to yourself with compassion, let your inner talk be compassionate also
- Focus on your strengths
- Do more things you LOVE often.
- Say "NO" to something that isn't a soul "YES"
- Let go of what you cannot control
- Stay far, far away from negativity
- Allow others to help you
- Write down three things you're grateful for.

The WOW moment- the transformation and what you can share with the world - Persist even when you feel the world is against you. Don't be afraid to change the scenery; if you are struggling, just do something you've always wanted to do because you never know who you meet or what experiences you will have. I had been in such a dark place, and packing my things was a cathartic experience, knowing I was moving to Canada. I'm living my best life, a life I've always wanted for myself...and have met my soulmate... now it's time to 'put-a-ring-on-it' Beyonce style!!

PS: You must dance a little in the morning before leaving the house because it changes how you walk into the world!

About the Author

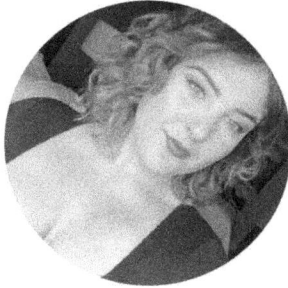

Dani Jasmine Middnedorp is a global traveler, an international bestselling author, a zoologist, and an animal scientist. She is studying for her master's in environmental management and is living in British Columbia.

Her zest and passion for life are expressed in her love for connection, taking a dip in the beauty Nature has to offer, and isn't afraid to let her vibrant personality shine.

She is expanding her soul journey by living each day as it comes, enjoys sitting by the campfire, and loves the full moon's energy.

Facebook: https://www.facebook.com/dani.middendorp.1
Instagram: dmiddz

-᠊ᢣᢣᢣ᠊→

Jill Natalia

"Grief is the response to a broken bond of belonging"
~ Toko Pa Turner.

The Gifts of Grief

When my best friend died suddenly in June 2022 I was in shock, disbelief and of course deep, deep grief.

Even now, in many ways, I still am.

Finding the right words to describe how many gifts this horrific loss has given me is vitally important and such a great opportunity for healing.

It is my hope that my lessons can be a small solace and offer a balm to the wounds that anyone who has lost someone dear to them may experience.

Simon has been in my life since I was 16 and he was 20. He was the eldest son of my first boss and was one of the most generous, loving, intelligent and wise souls I've ever met.

He is also the father to our 10 year old son.

Over the time since I received the news of his death there has been more anger, confusion, and exhaustion, in my life than I ever imagined I could handle.

But I have.

As C.S Lewis said: It wasn't just that his friend died, it was that the part of him that only his friend could bring out would never be brought out again.

I feel these words deep in my bones.

Who was I if I wasn't the person who Simon saw me as?

I had a choice; I could focus on the pain, or I could focus on the memories, the love and the laughter.

I could turn my focus to what the pain has taught me in order to help others go through this process.

In our culture, we are deeply unskilled in dealing with grief. We hold it at a distance as best we can, both in ourselves and in each other, treating it like the enemy of being productive and happy. There is unspoken shame associated with grief, it can feel dangerous and weak, there is a fear that we will stay in grief forever and become incapacitated by it. We fear we'll drown in our despair, or because it means falling apart in a world which values 'holding it together' above all else. But grief plays an essential role in our coming undone from previous attachments. It is the necessary current we need in order to carry us into our next phase of becoming. Without it, we may remain stuck in that area of our life, which can limit the whole spectrum of our feeling alive.

Grief is the expression of healing in motion.

Looking back through the dust and debris of this unexpected explosion I can see how imperative it was that I began to sift through the rubble to find the treasures amongst the grief.

And how the people around me have all changed and grown because of these gifts.

Gift one: Humility.

I am a counsellor. I have sat with many people who have lost children, spouses, parents and friends. I've heard their stories and encouraged them to keep going and invited them to look at things from a different perspective. I've helped to plant seeds of hope and supported them in their worst days.

After Simon died, I wanted to go back and apologise to all of my past clients.

I had no idea how debilitating grief is, how foggy your mind becomes and how incapacitated you feel. I also had no idea how hard it is to retain any information, how hard it is to make decisions, determine priorities and how hard it was to identify what I needed. I'm not an interventionist therapist so I don't tell people what they 'should' do. But in the days after Simon died, I needed someone to tell me what to do. I needed my supports in place to help me to move, eat, shower and rest.

I had to ask for help, there was no way I could do all the things that needed to be done and still take care of our son, work on and in my business and maintain a household.

Friends came out of the most unexpected places and surrounded me, in a way that let me surrender and start to heal. I am so grateful for their support. I see people who carry unprocessed grief for years (sometimes to their deathbed) and know that it can be transformed, but you can't do it alone.

Breathwork and Plant medicine were my main modalities for healing.

The type of breathwork I chose was Shamanic, or Conscious Connected Breathing.

If you have not heard of Breathwork before, a good place to start is your local healing groups. There are many different types of breathwork, so you might need to give a few of them a go to find your favourite. Ensure you find a trained well reputed practitioner to take you through this process: it's not for the novice.

My dear friend Kathy is a master practitioner and I was lucky enough to have her come to my house every two weeks to lead me and a small community group through Shamanic Breathwork sessions for several months.

It was exactly what I needed to start to let go of the heaviness of grief.

Healing doesn't happen while you are doing other things.

You need to make time and space for it. I'll say that again for those in the back as it's very important- **YOU NEED TO MAKE TIME AND SPACE FOR HEALING**.

Something else that I find is very effective to open up our subconscious and get to the root of problems is plant medicines. Cacao had already been in my life as a daily ritual and helped me to stop drinking caffeine. Part of my morning routine is to drink a cup of cacao with intention and inviting it into my body as a healing medicine, this feels both empowering and humbling. Let the medicines do their work....

I was lucky enough to have trained friends who could sit for me during therapeutic psilocybin and MDMA sessions. I became the person that was held instead of the holder. I let myself be seen in my grief and the surrender came from a place of no longer trying to keep it all together and not needing to.

I could actually feel the grief leaving my body, during a guided session. My mind created a scene where my heart opened and placed the grief on a little boat and sent it out on a calm lake.

Note: Just because this worked for me doesn't mean it's for everyone. Be discerning about what you decided to put into your body and make sure you do any psychedelics with a trained guide who has a calm nervous system and a non-judgemental attitude. Never take mind altering substances in a party setting or with untested medicines.

Gift Two: Courage.

I am no longer afraid of the things I used to spend so much time worrying about.

Freedom has risen inside me from these ashes exactly like the proverbial Phoenix.

The courage I feel when facing things that I would have avoided or stayed away from in the past are now where I spend most of my time. What I mean by this is I no longer play it safe, I no longer wait for things I want- I reach out and take them.

Engaging in civil disobedience has always been a bit of a habit of mine. I had joined the Extinction Rebellion group several years ago, and although I am quietly flying under the radar, my sovereignty flag flies high. I encourage others to speak up and let their voices be heard.

I have started two businesses that seek to empower people to find their voices and speak truth to bullshit. I believe in working with one soul at a time, I don't feel the need to jump and shout, in fact I speak very quietly and am quite still a lot of the time.

What I mean by that in practical terms is I feel called to disrupt business as usual, to eliminate the need for competition and comparison. Setting boundaries takes a lot of courage, I had to step into the uncomfortable world of saying what was ok for me and what wasn't and letting people down became a place I had to get used to in order to rest and recuperate.

I learned to say NO. I still say YES a lot, but got comfortable with NO.

I speak up, take up space and I ask for what's mine.

Gift Three: Belonging.

The difference between fitting in and belonging developed in a sad, but necessary way for me in the year after Simon died.

My relationship with certain family members has always been strained; I have never felt like part of the family. I left the country at 18 and was overseas for 28 years. After Simon died my family were not really able to support me, some even disappeared from my life. After feeling angry and abandoned I began to feel a huge wave of relief. I understood that not everyone deserves a seat at your table and you get to choose who you invite. Belonging is so different from fitting in, and I was tired of trying to fit in to feel accepted. I love the feeling of belonging, knowing that I can be my most broken and shattered self or my most shiny and radiant self and my circle will love me equally. The reprieve of not asking permission or seeking approval, having confidence in the knowledge that I am enough is life changing! I was able to fully embrace my core values of authenticity and belonging and when I am living within them life is calmer.

Gift Four: Strength.

After working on my emotional blocks and sorting out some of my stuff ('cause there's always more stuff) for the past 20 years, my mission has become strong enough to help others sort their stuff out.

By asking my clients:

What is getting in the way of your contribution?

What is REALLY stopping you from achieving your purpose?

Then saying "Let's look at that, I'm here for it, let's get stronger together."

By longing to make a difference in the world I have committed my life to creating community and connecting people to build an alternative economy of trust and service that builds better individuals who in turn build amazing communities. Taking control of my finances, not being afraid of making money and knowing my worth has been incredibly liberating. Strength comes in many forms, girls are not encouraged toward independence, but finding the strength to take care of myself in all ways has always been the greatest gift of all.

Gift Five: Comfort.

Simon was a trickster, he liked to keep everyone on their toes with sometimes shocking and inappropriate humour and quips. He was not always easy to be around and actually took pleasure in making people feel uncomfortable, especially me.

I didn't realise the impact this had on my children and myself over the years while I was still in it.

After Simon had a stroke in 2014 his wafer-thin filter became even more non-existent and his temper flared at any little inconvenience. Having a trigger happy housemate makes for tightrope walkers; we became guarded and afraid of saying or doing the 'wrong' thing that might set off an explosion in our home. We watched our words and became quiet, little church mice, not wanting to rock the boat.

It's taken a while to learn how to relax, but this gift of comfort has manifested as a feeling of relief and knowing that what others do has nothing to do with me, that emotions are just like the weather, not good or bad and ever changing.

I now have the perspective of being able to have consideration without taking things personally.

I knew when the people in my life who I expected to be there for me after Simon died weren't, it wasn't because they didn't want to be -

It was because they couldn't be.

Death is hard for some people to talk about.

That's why it's so important to get comfortable with it.

Gift Six: Connection.

Healing does not happen in isolation, it happens when we feel safe enough to open up and take a look at what has happened to us. To feel safe enough to speak our pain and not be judged. This is how we cultivate peace and deep belonging in our lives, by connecting to create community, and building authentic grounded relationships that foster our sense of self. From this place of grounded, aware presence all things are possible. When things are woven they are stronger. Connection takes time and intentional weaving; I am doing this in many ways, but mostly by putting myself around people who are also seeking connection. It is only through the connection to what we cherish that we can know how to move forward. In this way, grief is motion.

Gift Seven: Humour.

Laughter is ALWAYS the best medicine.

I remember the first time I laughed after Simon died.

It was on the day of his funeral.

We came home and the septic tank alarm was going off unexplained. I could feel his presence in this anomaly- loud, annoying and full of shit!

Then the rubbish bin wouldn't close, every time I pushed it closed it slid open again, it wasn't full and it didn't make sense.

I found these two things so funny and so like Simon…

It made me laugh so hard.

My friend Franc was with me, she saw the humour in it too. That night we had a big pillow fight with Rohan, rolling around on the floor laughing helped to shift the grief immensely.

Gift Eight: Love.

I thought I'd been in love many times before, but again I had no idea.

I met Andrew at a conference in May of 2021.

I wasn't looking for a partner, in fact I'd sworn I'd be single for the rest of my life and was completely unimpressed with the male race.

However, very soon after meeting Andrew I was overtaken by feelings I'd never felt before and when describing them to my friend I thought I must be sick; not eating, not sleeping and constantly light headed… She said I must be in love and I almost vomited.

It took me a long time to settle in and feel safe in love. Andrew and I were long distance for the first nine months of our relationship. I was happy by myself and felt in control, and focussed. I made all the decisions myself. I chose the music, the food and the surroundings.

I didn't know what it felt to be truly safe in a loving relationship, to be seen and loved exactly how I am.

And now I do. When something stuck can be released through grief, we are freeing up a greater capacity to love.

So I had to ask myself "What is the voice of me as a woman who is so deeply loved? How can I spread the love that is cultivated in my life like potent compost that can make for a fertile soil. How do I express myself to this man in a way so that he knows how deeply he is loved in return?"

We both have learned new ways of relating. Not from an egoic, wounded child or inner critic ways of communicating but a whole, healthy adult ways.

Rising from the ashes regaining strength, seeing myself as whole, well and complete.

When we remove the pressure of worrying about how we're going to show up (what we look like, what we will say, can we stay positive?)

and just actually show up then we can begin to relate in an authentic and vulnerable way that creates growth.

The other night while lying in bed I could hear the gales of laughter from Rohan as Andrew read him a book at bedtime. Andrew was doing all the voices of the characters and putting on a show for Rohan and it made me cry with the beauty of it all....

Gift Nine: Rest.

To learn how to stop and rest and not feel guilty or lazy has been the biggest challenge of my life. Sleep was evasive for quite a while, and when I did sleep my dreams were scary and confusing. But now I have developed a healthy sleep hygiene routine and am able to rest whenever I need to. From the outside grief may look like an expression of pain that serves no purpose, it is actually the soul's acknowledgment of what we value, we grieve the love we've lost but when we can rest fully and accept that love never ends we can find peace and in this place of peace we can truly rest.

Gift Ten: Patience.

When things come out of the blue we go into shock.

We think we have to push through and make decisions.

We don't.

Wait.

Take all the time you need.

Then wait some more.

I know it's hard and you want to move through the grief quickly, but don't.

Sometimes the fastest way through grief is by letting things be.

Turns out Lennon and McCartney were onto something- "When I find myself in times of trouble Mother Mary comes to me, speaking words of wisdom- Let It Be"

"Have you ever noticed how beautiful a person is after they've wept?
It's as if they are made new again by the baptism of tears."
~ Toko Pa Turner

About the Author

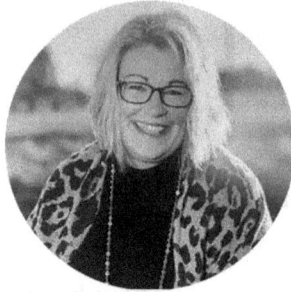

Jill Natalia is a vibrant and highly skilled facilitator, a Holistic Counsellor and Business Mentor with over 20 years of experience in Counselling and running women's circles. She is the mother to four amazing humans and is a partner to a magical medicine man.

She is the founder of Conscious Consulting NZ, Red Tent Aotearoa, and Red Tent Australia, offering Business Mentoring, Holistic Counselling, Strategic Development and Implementation.

Jill insists that diversity, equity and inclusion are the only ways forward and that competition is obsolete. She believes that focusing on collaboration is imperative to make the changes needed at this pivotal time. Her passion is authentic, compassionate Leadership Development and Assisted Therapies.

Email: jillnatalia@gmail.com
Website: https://www.jillnatalia.co.nz/
Facebook: www.facebook.com/RedTentAotearoaOfficial/

-ʌʌʌ→

Kim Sartor

'I am guided throughout this day making the right choices,' my gratitude card read.

I'm not so sure I agree. What a damn ride—this thing called life. If I'm completely honest, I have to say it's not been an easy one for me. Sometimes, I feel like I'm the happiest person on the planet, and then I feel like the saddest. What has changed me? On one end of the scale is the amazing birth of my children, and the far end of the scale is the breakdown of my marriage. I feel like I'm continually searching for *something more.* Not that my life is 'not enough,' personally, It's just not as fulfilling as I once imagined life would be. I feel like I need to find *ME.* I'm not lost, yet I don't know where I am or what I am supposed to be doing—deep down, an unfulfilled space exists.

I know I'm not alone in feeling like this, either. From a young age, I felt life was riding a rollercoaster with many ups and downs. As my life progressed, those loops and turns featured as experiences in many differing relationships, death, love, children, marriage, disasters, bliss, and so much more were bathed in light, and darkness. Yet, the suppressed moments and dark corners re-appear, deeply repressed emotions rise, and I continually push through it all. I am a happy and joyous person inside and out, and I have had an idyllic and happy childhood with a loving family, which is everything to me. Yet, I can't seem to fill a space inside me, not a hole, just a kind of emptiness.

I once imagined owning a little beach house. I've always loved the outdoors, the beach, swimming, the sunshine, the splashing of waves, my toes digging themselves into the warm sand, picking up discarded sea treasures– I adore all of this. I visualise a little seaside retreat where I could create a Cafe at one end, a little business just for me, where I could care for people and make others feel loved and nurtured. Create a cozy reading nook with fluffy throw pillows, plush blankets, and feel-good candles with a pop of colour. I would sit peacefully and sink into a petal-shaped armchair, disappearing from the world. I don't have a favourite book; I've read Wilbur Smith books that took me on journeys and crime novels as an escape that made me think. I've also enjoyed erotic and romance books, *blush*. I used to read much more than I do today. It inspires me to imagine filling this magical future quiet reading nook —filling this SPACE reading the books, maybe even books I've written myself (like this one you're reading now); others can sit there, too, in the reading nook, in my little 'Nimmy's Beach Cafe", sipping their Lattes and pouring their Pots of Tea, and nibbling homemade biscuits and heart-shaped double-layered cakes –my grandmother's recipe, of course–I used to love as a child. At Easter, I'd replicate our family traditions, and everyone will receive a marshmallow bunny, and my cake display will feature my Mum's awesome Sponge-cake and Pavlova. Maybe my future patrons, too, are on a journey to find themselves as they sit in my Cafe.

What do I want? I'm still deciding.

I sit here reviewing my past year. I'm ready to highlight my wins and focus on the miracles I've created within my life. I've moved into a Unit of my own, and my kids have completed their University studies and are embarking on their chosen careers and work. I enjoy supporting them in reaching for the stars. I blissfully sip my cuppa in my slouchy T-shirt in my own space on my own couch. LOVE IT!

But, still, *some kind of emptiness exists.*

It could be alignment. Hmm, I ponder, I'm not entirely sure. How else can I find my passion as an adult? I have spent most of my life looking after everyone else and bringing up three beautiful daughters, encouraging them to follow their dreams and have a go at whatever they want. Now they are adults, and I have more time for myself, I need to find myself.

It is nothing too thought-provoking, but a verse that comes directly down from my family has stayed with me through childhood to adulthood.

'A second-class car is better than a first-class walk.' I learned to drive in Dad's 4-wheel drive Ute back when we had the learner permit for six weeks— reverse parking between two 40-gallon drums, and excellent driving skills accumulated in the back paddock—Our family Falcon was clearly off-limits. My Father said that the second-class ride was better than the first-class walk. I now understand that the journey via the vehicle and not the everyday step that should be invested in. It's not each tear shed, each ounce of pain, each argument, every moment that defines me, it's the experience I've gained, the emotional choice, and the memories I choose to live with. It's not the quality; it's the ride.

There are others, as well, I have heard over time that have stayed with me.

'It's none of my business what other people think of me.' I struggle with this because I hate to think I have upset someone or they don't like me. As I grow older, I am learning to believe in myself, and another saying is, 'It says more about the other person than yourself on how they behave.' It's not a reflection of me but a reflection of them. I have one of those faces that tells on me, those moments when 'it's all out' and it's too late to bluff, and now I've changed the rules about how I let people treat me.

256

I have a shirt that says. 'If my mouth doesn't say it, my face will.' I've always felt I must school my face to ensure I don't give away my thoughts. I accept I have potential, and being treated like a fool–being lied to when I can see the truth is now off the cards for good. To the night, it's night permanently; to the day, it's bright, and the in-between is all that is space, *that emptiness* that neither side doesn't see.

At the age of 17, a boy I had dated was the driver of his car that had an accident and was killed–he was a beautiful soul I wish had not been taken so early, this is when I first felt an emotional hole start to tunnel out inside me. My first serious relationship was with someone good-looking and charming. Also, though he could make me feel really special, he had me doubting myself constantly, from my handwriting to how I was overweight, and I never felt good enough to be with him. I ended our relationship after three years in my final year of high school. I ended it, but I was heartbroken and still have doubts from that time that plague my mind. The tunnel became a hole, *a space.*

The deaths of my Uncle and my Grandfather within two months of each other was another devastating time. I can replay the phone call of when my Uncle was killed in an accident and then two months later, the phone call that my grandfather had passed. Then to watch my beautiful grandmother grieve her eldest child and her husband of 63 years was heartbreaking. She held on for another 15 years, ensuring she was around to see her

Great Great Grandchildren enter the world. She was a lovely person with a strong sense of self who took us all as she found us. There was nothing we as children, grandchildren, great-children, and great-great-great-grandchildren that would have her disappointed in anything we did. I witnessed the same tunneling *holes and spaces* created in others, too.

On a brighter note, fond memories of my 'Volleyball girls' from school. It was grade nine in high school in Rural Queensland, Australia, and my girl group—we initially decided to get involved with Volleyball as we had crushes on the boy's team. We then went to a school Volleybal Competition, and as the days and years passed, our hearts were full as crushes were realised into real relationships for some of my friends, I could feel their hearts pumping from my seat as they sat in their giggling and giddy ways next to 'their boys' on the bus road trips. " He looked at me," one of my girlfriends winked and whispered, looking over her seat at me. Some of those girls are married now to those very boys, now men, and I wonder if they are fulfilled or have some kind of *emptiness, holes, and space,* too?

Another real WOW life moment was when I left jobs when they were affecting my mental health—I didn't like who I was in that workplace and couldn't see how I would grow within that environment. The separation from my husband after 30 years of marriage, and our relationship was 34 years, affected both my work and mental state, too course. We grew up together, and we had three beautiful girls. We had done marriage counseling on several occasions, and we had talked, fought, glossed over things, and we both made mistakes, and ultimately, I wasn't happy, not just with the relationship but with myself. We did have a good marriage, and I never wanted to be divorced, I also needed to be true to myself. To everyone on the outside, we had the ideal partnership, but at times, neither met each other's needs. I wanted our girls to know they can put themselves first and still be a loving, caring person who has boundaries and is loved for themselves and by themselves.

What would it be if you could take impactful information to the world?

I want the world to know that not everyone has to agree with each other, and at times, it's okay to say okay, we can agree to disagree. Don't keep arguing your point if there is no moment in sight that you will agree with each other. Have a healthy conversation, but don't yell and insult others to make your point. I am not afraid to try new things. Still, I realise I fall back into the ease of life's daily processes and routines that have bound my life, and so many people have advice for me. I'm sure they mean well, but I read somewhere,' Never be afraid to try something new, remember, amateurs built the Ark, and professionals built the Titanic.' I love what I do, and my work, and I would still work because I like to be busy and have to own my own home. I want to travel and see more of Australia and parts of the world by myself and with my family, significant others, and friends. These things are all different and *new.* Doing new things in the new year of 2024 (like becoming a published Author, for example, what an opportunity!) may be the art of overcoming the *becoming–the process of finding ME!* Will it light that fire inside me for me to become me? As I love each day, I feel that balance and counterbalance are the vehicles I'm traveling. I feel like I've been searching for this elusive *balance.* What have I been passionate about? Getting through my separation and, ultimately, my divorce without too many scars and wounds to take forward from this point.

My main life goal is to find myself and be happy and healthy mentally, physically, and financially secure. This body I inhabit needs this balance and wholeness, too. It could be a case of stopping this bandaid effect, and I want to support my girls during their adulthood and watch them grow to be amazing women. I feel like in writing this; I'm making progress along my path, a cathartic experience to share and catapult myself onto the global stage, *blush again*. It's nice to know it is OK not to have it all figured out, OK not yet to have experienced balance, and OK not to be OK—it is the vehicle—the ride–the accumulation of emotional lessons—the spreading of my wings and noticing my natural beauty. That is my New Rule of wellness, too— noticing the beauty in each day no matter what's going on.

My other New Rule of Wellness: Be open to different ways or

remedies. Try to fix, not just use a band-aid measure or manage a health or mental issue. I want to get to the bottom of all this as well. I have chronic pain and other allergy issues, and although I have been to a lot of specialists and have had many scans, there is no finite answer. I am just managing everything now, but I hope to one day be mainly pain-free and feel well within myself. Fibro- was told by a physician I have fibromyalgia, then not too long later, I was told maybe I don't. This back and forth has weighed on me and plays with my psyche and body, affecting my mental direction, work, exercise, focus, relationships, and everything else. Maybe this Fibrosis is directed towards Perimenopause; maybe it's a hormone thing? For my overall health and Fibro, I am balancing life, Pilates, Gym, counseling, alternate therapies, chiro, acupuncture, massage, and elimination diet to control allergies and Graves. I feel it's a constant battle, and sometimes I just sit on my couch in my T-shirt and underwear, I often find if a fave song comes on, I dance around or tap my feet, sway and move my body, and sit and watch TV to block out the world.

Writing and delving into myself is refreshing, to externalize, and the project is all new to me, and to talk about myself as I'm doing today is bliss and freedom, maybe even *hole-filling*!

I've always thought I was searching for balance, but is it a case of being in the middle gradient of the extremes, or is it participating in things that I love or like to do? Is it balanced, or is it filling that emptiness, or is it none of the above? Enrichment that will cure the emptiness, it's not about filling a hole or being whole, its becoming fulfilled. 'A second-class car is better than a first-class walk.' Maybe enlisting Dad's quote is a strategy for my emptiness and balance, he provided me that answer so many years ago, and I've just realized it now.

I love the line— that resonates with me, "What if I fall, Oh, my darling, but what if I fly?" I had etched on a solid silver bangle for each of my daughters. I continually show up for my higher self; at other times, I feel like I'm fighting for space and solitude. Sometimes, I feel like it fills with fun and laughter; sometimes, it's somewhat complete with my own quiet time in my new unit where I've found happiness, but It's there, and I'm conscious of it. I'd like to call myself WHOLE, finding me while filling my buckets.

Reach out, I'd love a chat if my writing resonates with you…and one day, come for a latte at my Beach cafe!

About the Author

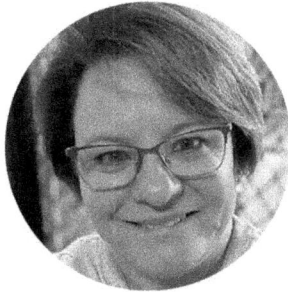

Kim, Nimmy to her friends, Sartor is courageous and a true health expert in her own self-development. She resides in Mackay Queensland and the proud mother of three gorgeous girls.

She embodies all things 'beachy' and works on creating her dream life and Nimmys Beach Cafe, others may think it's a pipe-dream, but watch this space as she is making progress along her lifepath.

She is on a wonderful journey to now find herself and find ways to spread her wings, and fill her buckets..

"What if I fall, Oh, my darling, but what if I fly?"

Email: kim.sartor@outlook.com
Facebook: https://www.facebook.com/kim.sartor.5
LinkedIn: Kim Sartor

-/\/\/\→

Dr. Heiraeth 'Reed' Sefra

I was named after a goddess of women, family, and childbirth. I've recently become a professional Spiritual Hygienist in my business, RaiseYour Vibes. I deal with the 'raw' power you can radiate to enjoy a fulfilled life and lift others. I feel I am an oasis for others to sustain their own life, to offer fertile energy to what lies beneath, and daily rituals for creating a routine that fosters self-care, energy renewal, and resilience. I embodied this throughout my life, but it wasn't always that way.

My ancestry is both Welsh and Portuguese, and I grew up in Texas and now live in New York. I've traveled to Australia and New Zealand, my two favorite places worldwide. I am still a Physician in Lower Manhattan, where I like to be called Reed by my friends and colleagues. I still love contributing to NYC Health, but my passion is energy work - what a mixed bag I am. By prioritizing spiritual hygiene, we can shield ourselves, change ourselves, and expand to defy our limitations—stop 'really struggling' and get out of 'exhausted, stressed, and depressed.' I only mention my medical training, from a professional standpoint, and merit for my life work focus. There is great evidence-based support that offers overall health and wellness as much as Emergency Medicine does.

My New Rule of Wellness: Say NO to Energy Vampires with mindful energy management.

New York is a happening place to be, and I call this amazing city my *home*. The Glasshouse Mountains in Queensland, Australia, is my *favorite* place in the world, and Queenstown, New Zealand, is my *spiritual* place. I mention these places because the significance of all three makes me feel about life today. I had three epiphanies in my life; these locations were where they occurred.

New York

New York, New York. I am a positivity Queen now. Nothing gets past me. " You can't always be that vibrant?" I get asked. Now, YES—Previously, NO! So what changed me?

I changed myself and had a few ideas about 'no more settling for less than I deserve.'

Making the space for amazing things to happen is the key.

Cleansing often and quiet boundaries are essential, offering yourself some peace in your hectic life, mindful management of life's details, and positivity all around you BY CHOICE. It's not about just thinking and feeling, its about cultivating the energy you desire to feel like, live, positively like, and sincerely become. New York did this for me.

So, luckily, I managed to get my dream full-time job in the medical field straight out of College—Not too far from my Fulton Street Condominium. I walk to work, and my colleagues are fantastic. I've been there for some years now and still love every minute. No horrible professional hierarchy like I had been told in the industry.

I also love my home. I cook, I exercise, I dine out, I see friends regularly, and I walk along Wall Street and visit the Titanic Memorial Park, and view the Brooklyn Bridge where I sit and sip my coffee. I love the history of New York and indulge in the vibe.

I also revamp my energy and protect my energetic-self on all levels—daily, which is how (organically) Raise Your Vibes was born. My focus is boutique bookings, and I have many professional and celebrity Realty friends here in New York via word of mouth I am booked 18 months in advance—how blissful.

I also love to travel; when I do, it's time off, well needed rest, and time to reboot.

And…now, it seems a published author!

Wootha

Glasshouse Mountains, Queensland, Australia. It is hot, tropical, and my favorite place to be.

My heart exploded there. I fell in love with an exotic man—a vacation romance–but he taught me to love again, an 'Eat-Pray-Love' moment. He was Eli-Arish, a tropical tree specialist who was in the area for a month with many College students on assignment for their cohort. I was also there for a month; it was the best month of my life so far. We laughed, we ate, we giggled in the hot tub, we sat under the Full Moon, and shared stories of loves lost, energy lost, energy gained—a real soul connection. We allowed it all to flow naturally and organically, knowing it would at some point come to an end—so blissful.

"You're a true Goddess," he told me on our last day together. What I learned from Eli was…everyone you meet and talk to isn't a coincidence. Listen to people; you will nourish them, and they will nourish you—just allow.

Arrowtown

South Island of New Zealand, Queenstown, is a little Lake district town, Arrowhead. Lake Hayes, my spiritual existence changed. It was Winter—puffy powder covered the ground, and the morning sun sparkled off the lake.

I met, clearly not by chance, the owner of the Airbnb where I was staying, and she asked if I wanted to join her in her daily early morning meditation ritual. Absolutely, I do!

The setting was idyllic, as was my gorgeous little cabin. My holiday rental cabin is a rustic log cabin with a claw-footed tub on the deck and a fire pit. The below Meditation I do each morning and night–has changed my life.

The Meditation

Find a relaxing position, either seated or lying down (anywhere, just comfortable).

Breathe in and come back to center.

Gentle close your eyes and shift your attention to your breath–in through your nose and let it out through your mouth, feeling your Lungs expand as you inhale and contract back when you exhale.

Set your intention for the day.

Pay attention to your body and really 'feel' each area, and give it permission to rest and relax for the next few minutes.

Your mind may wander off; use the breathe as your anchor and bring your attention back.

Let one thing today that you are proud of yourself for, and allow yourself to breathe the thought in for a moment; feel that feeling from the top of your head down to the tips of your toes.

Now think of something, one little thing that you can do today to bring in a renewed sense of yourself, one thing to increase your sparkle: maybe go to bed early so you can read that book?

Relax and enjoy the peace.

Now let's take a few more deep breaths together, feeling the expansion and the contracting back in as you exhale everything.

Give thanks for these few minutes you've taken for yourself, and in your own time, come back to where you are.

Being intentional and kind to yourself.

Gently open your eyes and intentionally enjoy the rest of your day.

***

So, what is spiritual hygiene? Why Protect ourselves from energy vampires – those people, places, and things that drain us?

I can help! There was a time when I was struggling with this — and it left me exhausted, stressed, and depressed. I have spent years exploring tactical strategies for daily rituals that can help safeguard our energy and elevate our performance in all areas of life — and I want to share with you.

Understanding Spiritual Hygiene

Spiritual hygiene refers to intentional practices to cleanse and protect our energy field. It involves creating a daily routine that fosters self-care, energy renewal, and resilience. By prioritizing spiritual hygiene, we can shield ourselves from energy vampires and cultivate a positive and vibrant state of being.

Forms of Meditation

The Foundation of Spiritual Hygiene: Meditation is the foundation for spiritual hygiene. It is a powerful practice that calms the mind, reduces stress, and connects us with our inner selves. Incorporating meditation into our daily routine creates a solid groundwork for emotional balance, mental clarity, and heightened energy awareness. Whether it's a five-minute guided meditation or a silent practice, make it a non-negotiable part of your day.

Setting Energetic Boundaries

Creating energetic boundaries is crucial for protecting our energy. Start by understanding how different people, places, and things impact your energy levels. Identify those that drain your energy and set clear boundaries to minimize their influence. This might involve limiting time spent with energy-draining individuals, avoiding negative environments, and being selective about the information and media you consume.

Daily Energy Clearing Rituals

This can be quite fun. Regular energy-clearing rituals are essential for maintaining optimal energetic health.

Some effective practices include:

- Smudging: Use sage, palo santo, or other cleansing herbs to purify your space and yourself. Allow the smoke to cleanse your aura, releasing any negative or stagnant energy.

- Salt Baths: Take regular salt baths to cleanse your energy field. Dissolve sea salt in warm water and soak for 15-20 minutes, envisioning the salt drawing out any negativity.

- Visualization: Envision a shower of pure white or golden light cascading down, washing away any negative energy and filling you with positive and revitalizing energy.

- Sound Healing: Use singing bowls, tuning forks, or soothing music to harmonize and cleanse your energy. Allow the vibrations to resonate within you, clearing any energetic blockages.

Mindful Energy Management

Become mindful of how you manage your energy throughout the day. Prioritize activities that uplift and recharge you, such as spending time in nature, engaging in creative pursuits, or connecting with loved ones. Practice saying no to energy-draining commitments that do not align with your priorities. Create a balance between work, rest, and play to prevent energy depletion and burnout.

Cultivating Gratitude and Positive Affirmations

Gratitude and positive affirmations are potent tools for maintaining high vibrational energy. Each day, take a few moments to express gratitude for the blessings in your life. Affirmations can also help reprogram your subconscious mind, replacing negative thoughts and beliefs with positive ones. Repeat empowering affirmations such as "I deserve positive energy and joy" or "I attract abundance and positivity into my life."

Surrounding Yourself with Supportive Energy

Surround yourself with individuals who uplift and support your energy. Seek out positive and like-minded communities, whether in person or online, where you can connect with others on a path of spiritual growth and personal development. Engaging in meaningful conversations and shared experiences with supportive individuals can significantly enhance your spiritual hygiene and overall well-being.

Prioritizing spiritual hygiene through daily rituals is essential for protecting our energy from energy vampires. By incorporating meditation, energy clearing, mindful energy management, gratitude, and positive affirmations, we can elevate our energy levels, maintain emotional balance, and enhance our overall performance in every aspect of life.

Become a positivity Queen! Once a month, I have this day I call "My Special Day", and you won't believe it when I connected with Dr. Dee, she said she has the same idea and practiced it for years. This is how I knew I was meant to be involved in her wellness book project. My special day is the 11th of every month, primarily because it is my birth date. On the 11th of each month, I take it particularly 'mindfully.', I am super sparkling, super kind, super flowing, super cleansing, and super supportive of my mind and body every month. I indulge in a portion of my favorite food; I relax a little more than I would on regular days;

I also learn a new skill (do a free little online course, or like this month, it's try juggling).

One Client testimony: When I lost all my excuses, I found my results.

Another Client Takeaway: Eat crap, feel like crap. Watch the news, feel anxious, Listen to all the rambling negativity in the world, and become very negative yourself. Go for a walk, feel relaxed, Listen to positivity, surround yourself with positive people, and feel inspired. Choose what uplifts you—you will automatically feel good, too.

I leave you with my journey in life with some sentences on living well. What is 'living well'? You decide for yourself! I have decided for myself! I have enjoyed expressing my 'my well-chosen words' here in this book—my legacy cemented with other astounding inspirations–how magical.

A life well-lived is a precious gift; hope, strength, and grace be with you always.

***

A Life Well Lived

What constitutes a life well lived?
Is it the money we accumulate,
The places we visit,

The Positions we hold,
The Accolades we win,
The Facebook friends,
The success of our relationships,
Or the legacy we leave behind?
~ J. Jos

About the Author

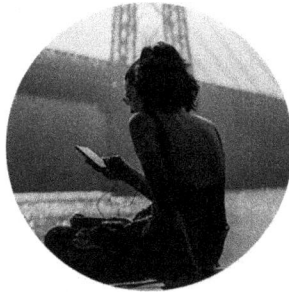

Dr. Heiraeth 'Reed' Sefra is a Physician in Lower Manhattan and loves her New York living.

Organically, her life unfolded to become a professional Spiritual Hygienist in my business, RaiseYour Vibes, a boutique service aimed toward enhancing that fertile energy to what lies beneath via daily rituals for creating a routine that fosters self-care, energy renewal, and resilience.

You will find her relaxing by the Brooklyn Bridge, sketching local scenes—even one day may have her work in a Gallery, traveling the world, learning and experiencing, and reading a good book.

Her message is embracing mindful energy management and living a well-lived life is the secret sauce.

Email: raiseyourvibe@gmail.com

-ᴧᴧᴧ→

Melanie Tambling

It was 2017. I had 4 children under 5. I was a stay-at-home mum with an amazing husband (who worked A LOT).

My days were filled with school runs, nappies, cooking, cleaning, and washing…oh the washing! I honestly didn't have any time to myself from the moment I woke, until I showered and crawled into bed each night.

One night, I happened to catch a glimpse of myself in the mirror…OH DEAR!! I was wearing old, frayed shorts and my husband's old gym shirt! This is what I had been sleeping in because comfort had trumped style. In fact, I had completely lost my style, my mojo and honestly, my entire sense of self. Don't get me wrong, I loved being home with my babies and they got to experience a very dedicated Mum. It was a wonderful chapter of our lives. But, after seeing my reflection, I was shocked and I immediately went on the hunt for new pyjamas! I set out on a shopping spree...wahoo! Unfortunately, my elation soon changed to despair. There were granny flannelettes and florals, animal prints and then the satin and lace types, with very minimal fabric. Not exactly suitable for wrangling 4 small children while doing all the Mum jobs. There just didn't seem to be anything practical and stylish to suit my needs.

So, the idea for ASHE was born...if I couldn't buy them, I'd design and make them myself! For the next 3 years, I kept my idea mostly to myself, only telling two people. But it kept creeping into my mind over and over. On a weekend away with a friend the name popped into my head- it's an acronym for my 4 daughters' names and it seemed perfect. I returned home and quickly got lost in my usual routine, but the idea was always sneaking into my thoughts.

A few years later I travelled Australia with my family and took this time to really consider where my life and career were headed. After many late-night discussions with my husband, we agreed that creating a sleepwear label was something that would take us out of our comfort zone, but worth pursuing.

I love the saying 'Why die wondering, just give it a go!'.

A few months into our big lap of Australia, our trip and lives took a different course than we had planned. Unfortunately, we faced two family tragedies. We put our family first and faced our challenges with determination and a whole lot of courage. We have become stronger as individuals and as a family unit. We always remember what a gift life is, and we are always making sure our life is on the path that we believe to be the best for our family. During this time of despair, I began saying to my husband 'Let's just forget about this sleepwear idea, it's too expensive, too risky, the outcome is so unpredictable.' But even while battling a serious medical issue and facing his own mortality, his response was always "this is the perfect time and if not now, then when? You have to keep chasing your dream."

Yep, I know, he's a keeper! Thankfully he has made a full recovery and is living a happy and healthy life.

So, we returned home, and I started my very own ethically and sustainably produced sleepwear label—Ashe. I naively thought it would be a simple process, boy was I wrong! After 2 years of late nights, highs and lows and a LOT of tears, Ashe finally launched as an Ecommerce business!!

Creating a sustainable brand, without compromising on quality is so important to me. I believe transparency and sustainability in the fashion industry are essential to mitigate the negative impact that clothing production has on the planet.

When creating Ashe, sustainability was at the forefront of every decision and practice, to produce and package our garments. Where possible, I have chosen to use natural fabrics such as Organic Cotton and Rayon. These fabrics are both 100%

biodegradable. We also use Shell buttons and Cotton labels...yep, that's right...no plastic is used! Organic Cotton is soft and breathable, making it the perfect fabric choice for sleepwear. Organic Cotton is grown without the use of synthetic pesticides or fertilizers, which can be harmful to the environment and human health. Rayon is known for its soft and silky feel, making it a popular fabric choice for clothing. The smooth texture of Rayon comes from its fine fibres, which are tightly woven together to create a lightweight and breathable fabric.

We only produce our garments in small batches to help eliminate waste. Small batch production can reduce the amount of excess inventory and unsold garments that end up in landfills. By producing only what is needed, small batch production can help to minimize waste and reduce our environmental impact. Furthermore, our small batch production supports a local business and community in Bali, by creating jobs and fostering a sense of connection and collaboration. We also create our scrunchies from offcuts of unused fabric, which helps to reduce waste while giving our customers a fun accessory to match their sleepwear!

Each garment arrives in Australia in a small bag made from the Cassava plant, which protects it during its journey to us. I then carefully pack each garment in recycled tissue paper, pop it into a Hero Mailer, and place a thermally printed postage sticker on it (all 100% biodegradable).

I'm so lucky to have our garments manufactured in a small, female led factory in Bali, Indonesia. This factory provides workers with a clean and safe workspace with adequate lighting and ventilation. Workers are there because they choose to be, there are NO child workers! Employees work for 8 hours each day with a lunch break, 5 days per week (workers even have a little nap during lunch time...such a Balinese tradition!). Overtime is offered, but there is no obligation to accept it. All religious holidays are respected, and workers are paid above award wages.

We also support the local communities by sourcing materials and labour from nearby regions. This creates jobs and stimulates the local economy, while also reducing the environmental impact of transportation. We work with so many local artisans who are incredibly talented, from our pattern maker and our printers, to our clever seamstresses, they all deserve to be treated fairly and with respect.

Now that Ashe is established, we continue to support many female led, Australian businesses like social media managers, copywriters, photographers, printers and designers. The flow on effect has a huge impact on females in business, particularly in regional areas. At the heart of Ashe is the reason I started working on it all those years ago. Ethical and sustainable practices are essential to everything I create at Ashe and something I'm extremely proud of.

But the Why? This is the most important aspect of Ashe, underpinning every decision I make.

The emphasis on the "Why?" reveals my motivation — the desire to empower women and boost their confidence and comfort through beautiful sleepwear. This focus on helping women feel good about themselves aligns with a broader commitment to individual well-being. It's not just about the product but the positive impact it can have on women. Integrating ethical and sustainable practices adds an extra layer of responsibility and care, not only for the customers but also for the environment and the broader community. It's a holistic approach that considers the bigger picture, and that commitment can resonate strongly with those who appreciate conscientious and thoughtful brands.

Feeling good in what you wear can be empowering.

It can inspire confidence, and a sense of control over one's life. This empowerment can influence various aspects of our lives. Fashion that focuses on helping women feel good goes beyond aesthetics; it becomes a tool for empowerment, self-expression, and overall well-being. When individuals feel comfortable, confident, and aligned with their values through their clothing choices, it can have a meaningful and lasting impact on their lives.

I frequently get to witness this mindset shift through my customers. I receive messages telling me that they've thrown out their daggy, old pyjamas and now love swanning around in their Ashe Sleepwear! They say they stay in it all day and even pop out to grab a coffee or do the school run without changing…What a life hack for busy Mums!!! This feedback is the whole reason why I created Ashe. I want women to feel comfortable in their sleepwear but ALSO feel a little bit glam and stylish. Our garments are perfect for taking on family holidays, especially on camping trips for a stylish dash to the shower block or a slow brekky outdoors.

It took a lot of time and patience to get our design exactly right.

I went through several rounds of sampling for each style. This involves sending garments back and forth between Bali and Australia marked with alteration and notes for the patternmaker. Each of these rounds costs thousands of dollars, but I was determined to sell a range that I felt had a perfect fit and I'd be proud to wear and recommend to family and friends (and now beautiful strangers). Printing our exclusive fabric prints also involved the same process. We trialled different techniques like screen printing and digital printing to make sure each print was an exact representation of what our artist had created. Again, I couldn't be prouder of the outcome we achieved.

I started this Label with absolutely no experience in clothing production and I naively thought that once I produced the garments launched online, things would run smoothly and garments would basically sell themselves. I couldn't have been more wrong.

Sometimes, I feel completely overwhelmed by the tasks and amount of learning still ahead of me.

While writing this book chapter, it's been nice to reflect on how far Ashe has come, how much I have grown as a business owner and the incredible amount I have learnt about Ecommerce. Who'd have thought I'd ever know what SEO, CTA and CRT acronyms are? I've put a lot of time into improving my copywriting skills, Shopify knowledge, Email Flows and of course, all things marketing. This is the BIG one, and I have realised that I really love learning everything about marketing! (Things I don't like are accounting and spreadsheets YUK!).

Another reason I have created this business is to show my daughters that they can do anything they set their mind to. I want them to see me living out my dreams! Knowing that at any time in their life they can start over, start late, be unsure, create change, try and fail and still succeed. Because having a dream and working hard to achieve it, no matter what the spreadsheets say, is always a success in my eyes.

When creating a product from the heart you need to believe that everything in life has a purpose and a lesson. You must be open to any opportunities that cross your path. I doubt myself all the time and I'm constantly pushed out of my comfort zone. Building a business takes a lot of time and energy and you need to be in it for the long haul. It's not easy, it really takes a lot of grit to keep plugging away behind the scenes. I have achieved things that I never would have thought I was capable of.

If I can live out my dream of creating and running a successful business then I believe anyone can do it! Remember what I said previously...'Why die wondering, just give it a go.'

About the Author

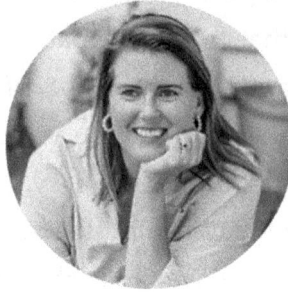

Melanie Tambling is married and has 4 beautiful daughters. She resides in Central Queensland on a quintessential lifestyle block with chooks, dogs, cattle and a veggie patch. Her family loves the lifestyle this provides. She has a Hairdressing background, but now devotes her time to her family and her Ethical Ecommerce sleepwear business. Melanie is passionate about helping women to feel great about themselves and adding a little style to their life. She loves supporting other female founded businesses, particularly those bringing products and services to Regional Australia.

In her downtime, you'll find her pottering around at home with a coffee in hand, cooking and spending time with her husband and children. She also loves to keep active by running and playing netball. She believes you can achieve anything with a lot of hard work, a little faith and a fair amount of crazy naivety.

Email: melanie@asheaustralia.com
Website: www.asheaustralia.com
Instagram: @ashe_australia

-∿∿→

Lauren Thompson

Lauren Thompson is a freelance writer of fantasy young adult books. She lives on the south coast of Victoria with her husband and dog, a beaglier named Sasha. She has a Bachelor of Arts Degree in Professional and Creative Writing and a Master of Arts Degree in Writing and Literature. Previously working with the Society of Women Writers Victoria (SWWV)

She writes under the pen name L. A. Thompson and has released 4 fantasy novels, three of which are part of a series called Isle of Dragons, first published in 2019—runner-up in the 2020 Readers Favorite Book Award. Future installments will be released in late 2023. The third book in the series, Isle of Dragons: The Ruler of Vansh was released in January 2024 and is now available on Amazon.

After dozens of sleepless nights at the keyboard and long discussions with my editor, and going back, editing and re-editing the manuscript until everything fit together like the pieces of a puzzle. My then partner shouted for joy that he could actually see me again, and he dragged me off to an all you can Japanese restaurant in celebration.

My third book in the Isle of Dragons series was a labor of love, in some ways, more so than the first two. It went through a number a changes, probably more than the first two did before publication. My editor guided me through the changes, encouraging me to go bigger with the story, adding more action, more characters, more conflict. "This is the third book in your series," she'd remind me. "It has to feel like it's on an even bigger scale than the last books." And getting the novel to that massive scale meant staying up late with a cup of tea (Okay, and the occasional Red Bull) until every scene, every word looked exactly how I wanted. The levels of sheer perfectionism around this book sprang from the pressures of making the third and final instalment in the trilogy come together in a way that made the storylines, character arcs and themes over the previous two books come together in a clear resonant manner for the target audience.

The Isle of Dragons series began with the concept of a girl who goes in search of a strange land to find her family, and meets many people who she finds a sense of connection and community with along the way. The third book ends with her finding the strength to save her world, through reconnecting to the people and parts of herself that she thought she'd lost. It mirrors so much of my own life and challenges with loneliness identity and finding my way forward. Fiction is a strange thing. You can write about dragons, magic and far off worlds, and it can be a great, fun escape, especially for children. But there always needs to be something that leaves readers thinking about the story, that helps them in some way. And one of the things I love most about writing is that you can explore deep universal themes such as grief, trauma and healing all having your characters create blasts of magic from their hands and ride on dragons. The weird mix of escapism and exploration of deeper themes is one of the main draws of genre fiction for people of all ages. Those days spent working and re-working this story were worth it, even though I had to chant the magic words "let if go" after the umpteenth rewrite (I would like to give you a solid figure at this but I lost count of the number of the rewrites I did after a while). The creation of all of my books came at a turbulent time in my life, and as I say goodbye to the time I worked on them, it also makes the end of one period in my life and the beginning of another.

At the time of the publication of the final book in my series and the beginning of the new year, I married my partner of two in a small service that consisted of a small group of friends and family. My husband is from the Philippines and I have found myself warmly welcomed by the Filipino community, and have to learn a different language, and I have come to enjoy cuisines that I had never had the chance to try before. The people from husband's family have shown me the warmth and acceptance of family. They have helped to give me the sense of connection that I had lost in the months prior to meeting my husband when I had lost my father to emphysema in May, 2021.

My mother had also passed away six years prior of emphysema, and my father's passing represented the loss of my immediate family. The same rhythms from the past repeated themselves. When I walked into his room in the nursing home he lived, he's eyes were closed, and his breathing grow labored, unaware of his surroundings. He was slowly slipping from the world. Six years ago, my mother had an emphysema attack, struggling to breath and unable to recognize her surroundings. She slipped into a coma that everyone from the ambulance workers to myself knew that she would never wake from.

He passed away in the middle of Covid lockdowns. I had a friend who was struggling with a chronic illness. I walked through everyday with a sense of loneliness and uncertainty, not quite sure of where I belonged anymore. My creativity and joy had faded, only to be reignited again after meeting the man who would later become my husband. The laughter, the shared food, and the small joy of walking on the beach in the cool summer air alongside him with my dog brought back the joy, security, contentment, and most importantly, hope, that I had lost. Little by little, step by step, I found my way out of the fog of grief and loneliness that I was lost in for so long. It was a time defined by a sense of deep loneliness and isolation.

Over the years since the loss of my family, I've built community with others who were also alone in some way or another. And while a sense of shared community is something that I've tried to infuse into all three books, this theme became particularly prominent in the third book, with characters forming relationships and finding connections in the most unexpected places during times when they need it the most. The third book explores the importance of community and finding a sense of community after loss and trauma. It is reflective of my own journey toward rediscovering community after the loss of my immediate family. Out of all the books, I've written, I'd say that the third book is by far the most personal and speaks to not only the grief of losing family, but of the joy and hope of finding people who can share in the highs and lows of life.

Throughout the book she is faced with the prospect of the world ending, and fights to keep her relationships, and the world from falling apart. When you're going through intense grief and isolation, it can feel like the world is ending. To feel like you're falling with no hope of getting back up again. But the people around you can reach down into that pit and pull you out if you allow them to do so. Jade's character ended up reflecting my own shifting understanding of herself and community. I wanted to create character for young readers whose main power didn't come from her strength, her ability to fight, or even her magic. I wanted to create a hero whose main strength came from her empathy, her and endless determination. A hero, whether they are a boy or girl, doesn't necessarily have to be great at kicking rear or punch lots of people to be a cool hero.

The series revolves around Jade, a girl who loses her place in society after her father is exiled and she has to go on a journey to find her family, all the while, expanding on her ideas of what belonging and family actually mean to her. She's always had interests and peculiarities that set her apart from others in her society, and when she lives her rather sheltered life to go and find her father, she meets other people who are also don't fit and are looked at with a mixture fear and contempt. She spends the first novel rejecting the things that make her unique for fear of not fitting in, only to embrace them, along with her expanded family. The journey that Jade takes is one of both self- acceptance and of finding community. It is also one of standing by our own principles and beliefs. Jade is told by everyone around her that it's wrong to use magic, and that she should follow along with corruption. Her mother died because she would not follow along with people looking to expand their own interests by praying in the vulnerable. At the end of the first book, one of the central antagonists asks Jade to help him at the expense of the people she's gained in her life. He offers the chance to regain her old life and live where she once did among the people who had mistreated her and her family. Throughout the first book, all Jade wanted was to find her father and clear his name so her life could go back to the way it was, to recapture a past that she knows deep down she can't. The first book revolves around her accepting that and moving on with her, while the 2nd focuses on her adjusting her new life and home. It's about her figuring out what her purpose is and how can protect her new home. In the climax of the third book in the Isle of Dragons, the main character is saved from falling to her death by someone who she had once considered family who she lost ties with due to their lives going in different directions. However, throughout the novel, they slowly began to reconnect with, remembering the bond they had lost. And at the end, they save one another. Genuine connection outside of the influences of their broader society and the problems arising in their environment that kept them apart for so long.

In the wake of my father's death, people came up to me at unexpected times and told me how he had helped them during a difficult time in their lives. These people ranged from old students to fellow war veterans. I heard more about the stories of how my father spoke out for the victim of abuse in Catholic schools, resulting in the firing and arrest of teachers in Victoria. He and my mother were eventually cut off from their local community. Mum had told me that was glad he had not stood down or compromised on the well-being of children. His friends told me how he had campaigned for them to have war service pensions and war widow pensions for the wives of friends who'd passed on. In life, he had stood for people. He had left a great legacy, but in the wake of his death, I became lost in the complicated time in which he passed. Adding grief into the already complex and fraught emotions that the lockdowns stirred in people, made a lot of emotions boil up inside of me. The last time the doctor went to see my father in his nursing home, he could barely talk. The emphysema and the Lewy Body Dementia that he suffered from at the time impacted his ability to speak, but the doctor told me that when she walked into his room, one of the first things he did was point to the first book in the Isle of Dragons series with a large grin on his face.

He passed away during Covid lockdowns, and anyone who lives in Victoria, Australia, would have vivid memories of the loneliness, isolation and sheer numbness that many of us felt at the time Over time, I would need think about what drove me and what I wanted to achieve in life. The answer came overtime, not in the middle of lockdown where my thoughts constantly rattled around in my head, but during the time that I spent with community, laughing, learning a new language and trying different foods. I had friends who were consumed by life in lockdown, and caught in the stress of caring for their family and themselves. We were all on autopilot, operating in survival mode, where connection was a luxury many did not have the time and energy for.

Before my dad passed, I treated being locked in my home the

same way many of us did in the earlier stages of lockdown. It was an opportunity to catch up on things I needed to do, to learn new skills and to create new things. Lockdowns meant sitting in front of the couch binging Netflix shows, or learning to bake or cook new dishes. For me, they also meant long hours sat in front of the computer typing out my novel, or later, marketing. Grief makes you lose sight of yourself. It eats away at your joy, your motivation; it robs you of all the things that make you who you are leaving you with nothing left to give. The slow pressure cooker that was living in lockdown began boil over. I was restless and agitated, and lacking in focus. I had lost the drive that had once kept me focused and sure of where I was going, with books and in life. At the time, I lived alone, and found myself caught gradually sinking into a sense of hopelessness. I was sinking deeper and deeper and could not draw myself out of it.

The story of what my father stood for has stayed with me. It is something that I carry in my life, and after his death, I have faced times where I had to ask myself if I would stay quiet when I saw people harmed by those in positions of power, or stand up for them. Even if it resulted in bullying and harassment from the organization I challenged, I reminded myself of why I kept getting back up after life (and the bullies), knocking me down, over and over. I did for those who didn't have a voice, for the people who were abused, underpaid and had their rights trodden on simply because of who they were. It's a fight that isn't over yet, but after feeling like anything I had to say didn't matter and no one wanted to hear my out, people are finally starting to listen. People in positions of power are taking notice. Someone I told about this issue once warned me to give up. They had fought a similar battle, and lost. They told me there was no way to win because everyone was corrupt. But I'm still climbing out of that pit, and still looking for the people who are not corrupt. I still have a long climb, but in my hopeless optimism, I want to think that I'm at least a little closer to reaching the top. Like Jade, sometimes I need someone to reach down inside the pit of lava waiting below and drag me down, but I need someone to reach down and let me know that I'm not alone, that they're there for me and they're not leaving.

The conflict in the final book may be aimed at a young adult audience, the themes of loneliness and hope in the darkest of times are ones that I believe can resonate with people of any age. Isle of Dragons has evolved from a story about a girl searching for a mysterious island where she uncovers secrets and meets people who help reconnect her to a sense of community while learning more about herself and her strengths while learning to move on from the life she had. The third and final book in the Isle of Dragons series is the culmination of years of work and the representation of major themes throughout my life, that include loss, defying expectations and reconnections. My hope for readers going into this series that they will find something in its pages and find just a little something that will bring them joy and maybe help them when they feel like they are falling.

About the Author

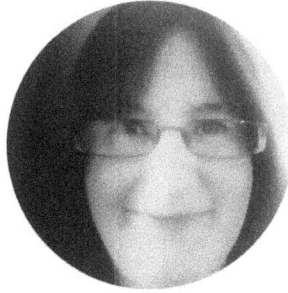

Lauren Thompson is a freelance writer of fantasy young adult books. She lives on the south coast of Victoria with her partner and dog, a beagle named Sasha. She has a Bachelor of Arts Degree in Professional and Creative Writing and a Master of Arts Degree in Writing and Literature. Previously working with the Society of Women Writers Victoria (SWWV).

She writes under the pen name L. A. Thompson and has released 3 fantasy novels, two of which are part of a series called Isle of Dragons, first published in 2019 — runner-up in the 2020 Readers Favorite Book Award. Future installments will be released in late 2023.

She has written a standalone novella called The Prince and the Witch.

Website: https://la-thompson.com/

Where to buy my books:

https://www.amazon.com/Isle-Dragons-1-L-Thompson-ebook/dp/B0B85XJS29

https://www.amazon.com/Prince-Witch-L-Thompson-ebook/dp/B09YYKSYRW

-vvv→

Barb Whitfield

Be Well Be You

I've always felt that I've been given a special gift to share with all that cross my path.

Something that was given to me way before my birth, I see and feel things that others seem not to notice, I hear the unspoken words from people when they are communicating with me.

The eternal flame in my heart tells me that we are all connected, and everything happens for a reason. The universe guides me where I need to be and shines my light bright for those that may benefit from finding me.

When I have my first session with someone, I see their body language, how they sit, walk, how they breathe, if the light in their eyes is bright or if they have lost their way. All these things leap out at me and tell me this individual's story.

I was given a piece of very useful advice a very long time ago that I like to live by and share.

Always accept what is and build on the positive.

Over the past several decades I've met and been invited to join so many amazing individuals on their wellness journeys. The strength and determination of a human being never fails to astound and amaze me. Please read on and join me sharing a snippet of an inspirational being.

Conies Journey

I feel very blessed and fortunate the day that Conie telephoned me and invited me into her life to assist and support her. Conie explained to me on the telephone that her doctor had recommended that she contact me. I asked why her doctor had suggested this and Conie said that she didn't want to leave her home and would I come to see her. Her doctor had written a letter to give to me and we agreed on a day and time the following week.

Knocking on Conies door a few days later, I watched as she slowly approached the door, using the aide of a wheelie walker. Her body was slumped forward, shoulders stooped. Eyes were dull, listless, her hair seemed unbrushed had looked like it had not been washed for several days. When she spoke, it was very slow and drawn out as if it was a huge effort just to talk.

Her breathe was shallow and quite noisy.

Sitting at the kitchen table I read the doctors letter, it included a clearance for her to do some gentle physical form of exercise, a list of medications that Conie was taking, all her current and past medical history and a list of other allied health professionals that she was seeing including a physiotherapist, a dietitian and a psychologist.

Conie was in her mid 40's, weighed 140 kilograms, was 152cm tall, suffered seizures if her blood pressure increased, had numerous current medical challenges including diabetes, breathing concerns (lack of lack capacity), sleep apnea, arthritis, osteoporosis, chronic fatigue, and mental health unwellness.

I simply asked what her goal was, what did she want to do with her future, she looked towards the floor. Conie said she wanted to be able to walk outside without feeling that people staring at her due to her weight, to attend church again and be able to walk freely and unaided. I found out that the last time she had been out of the house was over 2 years ago and she felt like everyone just stared are her because of her size so she stayed home as it was her haven, a place where she felt safe with her husband.

Conie explained that she always had a dislike for exercise because it hurt, was boring and she couldn't do it by herself as she was not motivated.

I suggested that if I came to her house twice a week and wrote some very simple things for her to do and if I rang her the other 5 days at 11am to support her see how she went with the program, did she think that would be achievable? She said yes and we agreed on the days and times I would come over.

On the first visit I arrived with a monthly chart with the different days of the week to pop on her fridge. She was to draw a smiley face if she did her tasks on that day. If she didn't do them simply to write why, Eg: to tired, not well etc. I bought a large and small ball and gave them to her.

For the first 4 weeks her program consisted of sitting at the kitchen on a chair and bouncing the big ball and catching 10 times with 1 hand and then the other (with rests in between).

After 4 weeks I added walking around the entire internal walls of her home first 1 way and then in the reverse direction.

Each 4 weeks as Conies health and strength improved, I changed / or added simple movement patterns to it. Some sitting, others standing holding the back of a chair.

Each session concluded with a breathing meditation to increase Conies lung capacity, reduce her anxiety, improved her mood, and assist her to find her own inner peace.

After 3 months Conie started to notice that she was feeling better, her body was moving with less pain, her breathing had improved, and she only missed 1 or 2 session a week when doing

her program by herself. Her doctor, dietitian was physiotherapist were all happy as she had lost 6 kilograms.

After 6 months, Conie was excited to purchase a new pair of training shoes as her old ones were now too big for her feet. 12 kilograms had disappeared from her body and was starting to be replaced with muscle. The program included seated simple movement patterns with homemade weights (rice in pillowcases), small squats holding the back of a chair and walking on a walking machine and wall pushouts.

Each time I went to her home or spoke to on the telephone, it was like she was discovering herself again. She was happy and her body was responding happily to movement, breathing and meditation. Conie was a breath of fresh air to support and motivate as she was seeing the results and feeling so good. I suggested that the following week we could included a walk to the park (it was 3 x doors away) in her program. To my excitement she said yes, let's do it.

Over the next 6 months Connie continued become stronger and improve her health, she was an inspiration. She no longer needed to walk with an aide, she had a bounce in her step, her eyes had a fire of determination and she kept saying "I'm back,

I'm back". I asked her what that meant, she said that she had given up on life so long ago and just before our first meeting her she had been contemplating taking an overdose of medication as she felt as if her life was just never going to get better. Conie thanked me for everything that I had done for her. I explained that I can only support, motivate and assist but she had done all the hard work with her sheer determination. She was an inspiration to all. She gave me a hug. I could feel her happiness in every fiber of my being. I thanked the universe for my gift.

It was heading towards the 1-year anniversary of my time with Conie, the majority of her program was now done in the park with the exceptions of her interval training on the treadmill and her breathing meditation. I still visited her twice a week to supervise and adapt and change her program as she continued to improve. I had stopped my support telephone calls. Conie had not left the house except with me to the park, I suggested we go for a walk around the shopping center the following week. I reassured her that she was not the same individual that I had met 12 months before, she had lost over 20 kilograms, was a strong and confident female that could do anything that she put her mind to. I heard her take a sharp breath in; I was expecting her to say no. To my amazement she said yes, let's do it.

Five days later when I picked up Conie to go for a walk around the shopping center, she said that she had already walked to the park herself and completed her program. I congratulated her on how far she had come in 12 months. I felt that she was now self-reliant to do her program without me. I acknowledged to myself that our time together was nearly over, and I was so happy that she was now ready to take on the world. At that moment I felt truly blessed and felt so much gratitude to have been a small part of Conies journey.

As we got out of my car at the shopping center, I noticed she was a bit nervous. I started to chat with her about what shops may have changed since she was there over 3 years ago. Once we were talking and walking, she relaxed and stopped to look at each shop. Then she started to say she wanted to make a hair appointment for next week and do we have time today if she got her fingernails done. I smiled as sometimes it's the little things that can mean so much if you've been away from society. As we got both of our nails done, I said 12 months ago there were 3 goals that she told me that she had wanted for her future. Two of them had been achieved; the feeling of being able to walk outside without people staring at her and to walk freely and unaided. Maybe it was time to do the third one and attend church again.

Connie said she had forgotten about that goal. Her pastor had been visiting her at home every week for the past 3 years. She said she would have to go shopping for some new clothes as all her church clothes were way too big for her now. I explained that I had time, so we went shopping. I don't think I've ever seen anyone so excited about trying clothes on. We did 5 shops and she got 4 new outfits. She was smiling from ear to ear. She felt confident in herself internally and externally. Sometimes it's the internal battle that we have with ourselves that is the hardest part. Finding someone that will support and assist you to take the first step can be the most difficult.

I saw Conie for two more weeks after that and all she could talk about was how she felt going back to church and walking in unaided. I explained to her that she no longer needed me, and it was time for me to assist and support another human being. As her program would need to continually be changed to challenge and support her wellness, I gave her the details of another highly qualified health professional who would assist her on a 1 to 1 basis in a gym.

I still catch up with Connie for lunch every now and again. At the time of writing this is happy and loving life to its fullest.

I have an attitude of gratitude that the universe guides me where I need to be and shines my light bright for those who may benefit from finding me.

I was 12 years old when my mother passed over, in the week beforehand, she said to me, "Always accept what is and build on the positive." Throughout my entire life this has been the guiding piece of light that I've followed.

Thank you for taking time to read my chapter, I'd love to offer you a free Breath Work information sheet that will assist sleep soundness and calmness. You will find my contact details in my bio.

If you feel you that yourself or a family member could benefit from seeing me, please reach out. I would feel blessed and honoured to assist you in any way that I can. Either face-to-face or via the simple technology of Zoom.

The first step can be the hardest.

Until our paths cross again, blessings and safe travels. Barb

About the Author

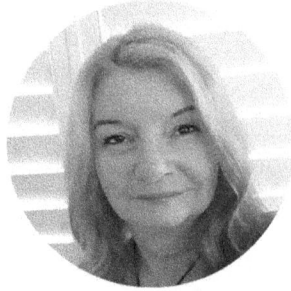

Barb Whitfield created and founded 'Be Well with Barb' over 35 years ago. She comes from a health science background that spans over 4 decades.

Barb is the designer of several national training programs, including 'It's Your Life Be Active,' 'Ageing with Vitality,' and 'Breath into Life.' Barb has received several national awards for her contributions to the health and wellness area, and she lectures nationally and internationally.

Her dream is to heal the world one person at a time. Being down to earth and an eternal optimist, she thinks outside the box, passionate about assisting individuals in finding their quiet calmness within.

Website: bewellwithbarb.com.au
Email: barb@bewellwithbarb.com.au
Facebook: www.facebook.com/bewellwithbarb

-∿∿→

Angela - ANON - Z

Let's do this thing!

This is the story of Angela and Zeke; I am Angela. A story that will take you from a magical, serendipitous relationship to a most tragic ending—To Hell and back!

I leave my house with 200 unread text messages. Yes, I'm a mess. A heavy pain sits in my chest and feels like it will never leave— A pain that aches and jabs, with a certain kind of numbness and a strange creeping-up-my-throat-sensation that rises and falls. The *dings* of inbound emails that I also can't face increase the intensity of my existence. Funny though, I've come to like myself like this: it's my new normal.

On my way to the studio, I listen to the new song by AR in my car, and my current energy resonates with the words; then silence fills me. The sound of silence holds everyone's secrets.

I am an acclaimed artist, a songwriter, and a literary writer—as a side gig, when I feel like it, (which seems to pay the best), I get lost in my reverie of writing.

Another *ding* on my phone. *'Did you like your Uber Eats order?'* The app wants me to leave a positive review. One day, I will again cook for myself; I just can't deal with thinking about food or, anything but Zeke! I wrote a melancholic ballad about love lost in the entangled web of love and heartbreak, the mess of my beloved Zeke, and the echo of our dream. I feel that I am still an 'entangled particle' in the mess of my life and so sensitive to his energy, no matter where he is. I know it's so evil of me—but would I rather he had died? I can't get this thought out of my mind.

Dead.

Guilt plagues me for continually thinking this. I feel I would be able to grieve his departure and grieve the loss, but knowing he is living another life in another part of the world with another person is killing me. I am the one that is dead inside.

DEAD.

Maybe it was me who died?

I can't stop thinking how I'm overthinking that too—how painful it is for others to be around me, with all my *deadness*. I do not foresee any part of me 'working through this phase' (as some of those 200 SMS messages suggest I will do).

I get up daily and convince myself, *let's do this thing,* then I chant to myself aloud in a melodic tone that I'm most pleased with—catching the High-C note, "Let's do this thing."

I look in the hallway mirror and catch my reflection dancing to my song, coffee in hand. Some days, coffee splashes on the floor; others, the liquid gold makes it to my lips and soothes my pain.

"Let's DO THIS THING CALLED LIFE TODAY." Then, Rinse and Repeat daily for the working week.

Then, Saturday arrives, and I dream.

My beloved Zeke is beside me, stroking my long, thick hair; he loves curling the ends around his Pinkie. I lean over and sip my morning coffee, so delicious as he had just made it for me, made with love as he does each morning. No words are spoken; we smile and end up giggling. I feel the gratitude flowing through us both, and I feel his energy. And when we are physically apart, spiritually, we are always united, for love transcends space and time. Nothing is ever missing.

My eyes flash open.

Reality hits.

I'm alone—just *a dream.*

I used to cry for many years, but now my tears have long gone, and my tear ducts are parched and dehydrated, just a Desert space now.

Forgiveness— I remind myself. 'I need to forgive,' I say to his oversized portrait I stare at daily, the one I painted of him that hangs on the largest wall in my space.

'Stop focusing your energy on past events, for life is too precious to waste,' my mother's voice echoes and ricochets around the few brain cells I have left.

'You create your reality, Angel, by what you think, dream, and imagine.' says my best friend as she calls each Saturday morning to check in with me.

I know I am living inside my self-absorbed head. I can't find a way out. I *think* of an idyllic life with Zeke. I *dream* of him wandering through the New York City streets and finding me again. In my mind, I see him walk along down near my gallery, down Allen Street, and come around Orchard Street, see me sitting in the Froth cafe, smile at me, nod and winks too, and kiss me like he always did, and joining his fingers together making that well known 'heart' shape with his hands. (The image in Dr. Dee's book here resonated with me instantly). At other times, I also *Imagine* him sneaking a 60-carat diamond ring into a stemless Waterford crystal glass of French champagne– *think, dream, and imagine!*

My life had been so magical, such the most amazing serendipitous relationship I've experienced with Zeke for many years. We took carriage rides through Central Park, sat in A-rated cafes, and chatted as if we lived in our little world of bliss. I supported his passion for Crypto investments and the adventures he dreamed of taking. The day I painted his portrait was serendipitous, too; time lapsed, and the sitting seemed to last for hours. I sketched and painted; we had a few breaks, walked in the sun, swam in our pool, and ate grapes on the sundeck outside our bedroom at our Villa.

"Who has a villa in the CBD of NYC? Zeke DOES!"

"You are the luckiest girl alive," My BFF told me. "Zeke has it all."

Today at the Gallery, Jennifer lit a fire under my butt.

Jennifer is the Curator at the Gallery. I call it *MY* Gallery, but it's not mine; I've just worked there for many years, and this is where I first met Zeke eleven years ago. He walked off the street one sunny Spring morning, his nose trailing the coffee scent from the sidewalk to our Gallery's little boutique cafe with the most delicious freshly ground coffee. Irresistible are the aromas,

"Irresistible" is what he called to me, referencing and gesturing that *I was irresistible,* not the coffee.

"ANGEL!" yelled Jennifer from the far corner, bringing me back into present reality.

"Get with the program we have a Gala to set."

Today, we have a Gala exhibition opening with a famous guest vocalist, resident artists, myself, and the excellent Jennifer. She never fails to inspire me. I've never met anyone whose voice excites me more. She sings with power, tone, pitch, and control, just beautiful, but no one would know that she has this ability. I caught her singing in the cafe area when it was closed while she stacked the chairs. She thought she was alone, and one day, she was a little tipsy and belted out a Disney song.

"What an amazing set of pipes!" yelled out another tipsy artist, knocking over a canvas with his exaggerated arm gestures.

Another afternoon a few years before Zeke left, a vocalist was booked at the Gallery for a champagne evening but was a no-show, "the show must go on," Jennifer voiced calmly, and ended up singing the entire set herself. " No problem at all!"

Jennifer is confined to her wheelchair due to a rare genetic condition where her hands and feet never formed adequately. She hasn't stood a day in her life, but her personality stands tall. She loves her pool exercising, particularly after her last round of surgery over 12 months ago; she has developed an affinity to water and all things aqueous.

"I can walk in the water and even swim like a mermaid; I am Aerial!" She then belted the score of Disney's The Little Mermaid, "I identify with Aerial so much."

Jenifer is the most inspiring woman. When I'm around her, I seem to forget my numbness and pain momentarily. " You are courageous and real," she tells me when I'm the most glum at the Gallery.

"Oh, for Disney's-sake, Angel, Knock-knock-tick-tock," she gestures at her forehead and Cartier watch. Little did I know that today would be my life's most memorable and best day.

My Mantra has been: Think, dream, and imagine!.....think, dream, and imagine! I chant over and over and over. Helps me pull the brakes on my self-destructive thoughts. It's not easy, what do I want?

I've been doing meditation daily, the above-entitled, and I want to share it with you. It has been very healing for me, and I feel it's the answer to many 'unanswered' emotions and is responsible for the metamorphs of energy in me.

Meditation for healing:

Just imagine you are surrounded by light, green healing light; cleansed, healed.

Take a deep breath, and as you breathe, close your eyes and any thoughts or concerns that may hinder your healing. *FEEL, SENSE, IMAGINE.*

Greenlight fills every cell, skin, and energy field with light, and any darkness is lushed out with the light. With each breath you take, your energy expands until it fills the room, the whole space around you now energizing you and stepping into the truth of who you are — as light beings. Be fully aware of this green lightal around you — the energy of healing. Anything you have been holding onto–anything that no longer serves you, let it flow down to your feet and back into the earth. Make an intention to let go — feel the energy move through you, now allow this energy to move down and anything that you have been holding onto, just allow it as it doesn't belong to you anymore and is no longer a part of your consciousness, no long your path. The energy of your gratitude and thanks brings you great joy and happiness, the light of abundance and blessings. *Think, dream, and imagine*– open the doors of your heart, places you have stored away information and energy that is not to you anymore–and let that energy go — imagine it flings away–think, dream, and imagine your ultimate dreams coming into reality. By closing the doors to the energy of the past, your Karma is healed. Greenlight surrounds you— *think, dream, and imagine*—open your heart to receive and embrace it with every cell.

***

Little did I know that today would be my life's most memorable and best day: The Gala was buzzing, the Gallery filling, the Champagne flowing, and smiles on everyone's faces.

"Angel…..My Angel," a familiar voice echoed. I froze. I listened, my wide 'bug-eyed' look frozen, both eyes open in an intense stare.

"Angel…. My Angel," I heard again, louder this time. I shook and nearly collapsed, it was Zeke. He stood before me, and I blinked. "WHAT?" I squeaked out.

He took my shaking hand in his, and I instantly calmed. "What are you doing here?" I managed to blurt out. A million thoughts ran through my head. I had imagined this moment repeatedly; the next time I saw him and what I would say, I was suddenly mute, "WHAT?" I said again in an even softer voice.

"I've made a terrible mistake', that's all he said, well, maybe, that's all I heard. My eardrums received his deep, low-toned sound waves; his frequency matched mine. He was talking, but I couldn't hear. I melted and froze at the same time. I simultaneously combusted and was reborn. His words hung in the air, the sunlight shone brighter, the coffee smelled richer, and the ever-increasing crowd seemed to part and flow around us, such a vibrant green light surrounded us.

Was I imagining all this?

Was he standing in front of me?

My mind catapulted back to many happy times, amazing times, and magical times—Sitting in the garden of my apartment sharing a conversation, giggling in the back of the cinema, soaping the loofah in the bathtub, and splashing the water all over the floor, overflowing the liquid soap in the outdoor spa at a holiday rental—the suds spilling all over the back patio. Amazing times that I watch and rewatch like my own home movie clips, but in my mind.

Is he standing and holding my hand?

Will my eyes soon flash open for my painful reality to hit again? His lips stopped moving.

He just held me. The resonating frequency and connections ebb and flow. I feel the sunset and the moon rise, and the seasons come and go. I feel the weathering of the storm and smell the wildflowers of summer. I feel sunshine return to my shoulders and smile. He smiles back. He feels my muscles start to relax.

More thoughts race: We had so many years of amazingness. I still can't figure out what happened, why he left, who he left with, and where he went. We were so perfect for each other, so good together, everyone said, " Angel and Zeke, what a made-in-heaven couple."

I now cast *all that* far from here, far away from this moment. All those thoughts that had become my life– vanished or combusted, I'm not sure which.

Acceptance is the key to inner peace. At times, we must accept things as they are, as they appear, and as they turn out. I have slowly learned there is no point in changing what is beyond our control.

Zeke now looks at me deep into my soul.

We smile at each other with no words. We suddenly giggle as though no time has passed; I feel his energy and are always united; the sound of my silence has broken; nothing is ever missing; it lives within. I know my voice is powerful, and my message and voice will shine through anything. (If my story is the only thing you read today, I hope it offers you comfort and hope for everything you may be dreaming of. Don't give up on yourself; you are also wonderful and worthy of love.) I was honored to be asked to be involved with such a powerful publication as The New Rules of Wellness, and this is my new rule. I wish the world to hear my voice, thoughts, and feelings and that my past heartaches have been remedied with the pure energy of acceptance.

I see Jennifer and the Gallery Guests gather around us. Zeke hands me a stemless Champagne Flute; he is holding one, too, everyone seems to beholding one, the most effervescent pale gold bubbly with a pinkish glow. I see something in the bottom of the glass reacting to the afternoon Summer light— a complex prism rainbow effect— I can see each color of red, orange, yellow, green, blue, and violet, and time stands still. The Diamond Ring was so brilliantly sparkling in all its glory; the bouncing light caught my eye for what seemed like an eternity.

Zeke's eyes were offering some refraction, too. He is whispering to me, but I again cannot hear. I hear the crowd roaring behind me and Jennifer's voice….and the noise of my thoughts: *think, dream, and imagine!*

"Let's Do This Thing!" His smile was infectious, "I've made the most terrible life judgment, Will you Marry me, my Angel?"

"Let's do this thing!"

About the Author

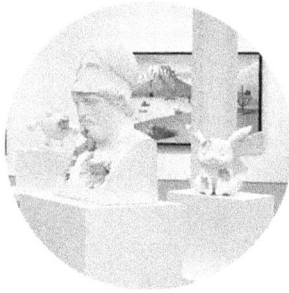

Angela is a resident of Manhattan, an acclaimed artist, a songwriter, and an award-winning literary writer. Her writing fodder comes from her life experiences and connections, and as a whole, she is a hunter of words.

She has a hunger for all things unwritten and is on a hunt for all things begging to be created into a song.

You will find her on a far-off beach with her husband Zeke, sipping espressos and watching the sunset over the New York skyline, or curled up with a good book—in reverie.

She will be in her Gallery in Lower Manhattan—welcome for coffee and some Daniel Arshams art!

"Every artwork that will ever be made is out there already, the materials just have to be brought together"
~ John Delorian Tells All.

www.ingramcontent.com/pod-product-compliance
Lightning Source LLC
Chambersburg PA
CBHW060025030426

42334CB00019B/2191